The Face of Madness

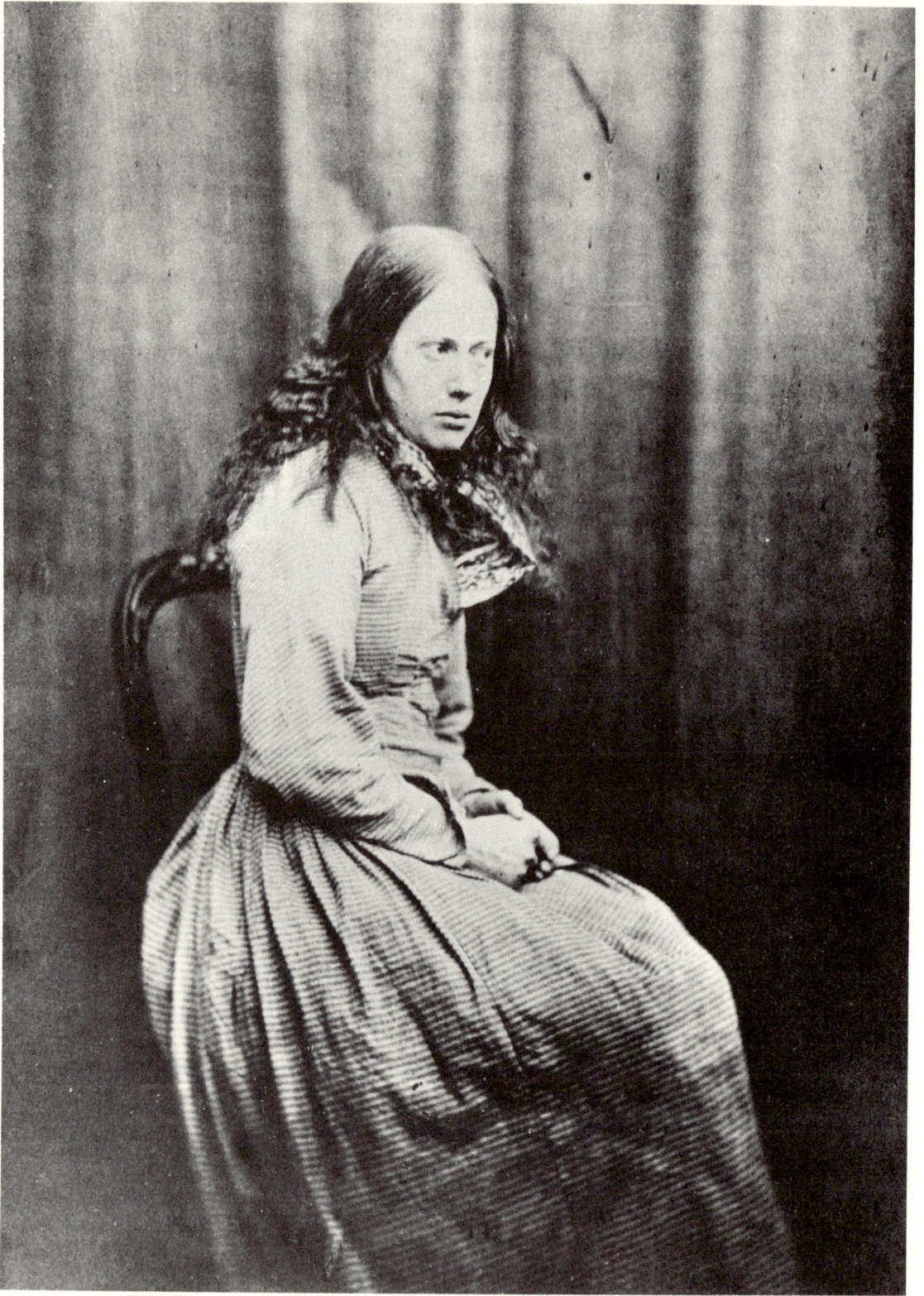

The Face of Madness

Hugh W. Diamond

AND THE

Origin of Psychiatric Photography

EDITED BY SANDER L. GILMAN, PH.D.

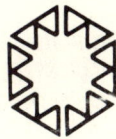

BRUNNER/MAZEL, *Publishers* · New York

Library of Congress Cataloging in Publication Data

Main entry under title:
The face of madness.

 Includes bibliographical references.
 CONTENTS: Carlson, E. T. Introduction.—Gilman,
S.L. Hugh W. Diamond and psychiatric photography.—
Diamond, H. W. On the application of photography to the
physiognomic and mental phenomena of insanity. [etc.]
 1. Photography in psychiatry—Addresses, essays,
lectures. 2. Psychiatry—Early works to 1900—Addresses,
essays, lectures. 3. Physiognomy—Addresses, essays,
lectures. I. Gilman, Sander L. Hugh W. Diamond and
psychiatric photography. 1976. II. Diamond, Hugh
Welch. On the application of photography to the
physiognomic and mental phenomena of insanity. 1976.
III. Conolly, John, 1794–1866. The physiognomy of insanity. Selections. 1976. IV. Gilman, Sander L.
[DNLM: 1. Face. 2. Mental disorders—History—
England. 2. Photography—History—England. WM11 FE5
F13]
RC455.2.P5F3 616.8′9′0028 76-23170
ISBN 0-87630-132-4

Published by
BRUNNER/MAZEL, INC.
19 Union Square West, New York, N.Y. 10003

TO

Marianne Horney-Eckardt

PREFACE

The use of photography in psychiatry is today a common practice. Whether to illustrate textbooks or to function in personality testing, the photograph is an integral part of the psychiatrist's tools. The present monograph presents all of the clinical photographs of the first psychiatric photographer, Hugh Welch Diamond, as well as his paper on the use of photography in the treatment of the mentally ill.

The photographs, all without case studies, are preserved in the archives of the Royal Society of Medicine (London), the Norfolk Record Office (Norwich), and the Royal Photographic Society (London). I am indebted to these archives for permission to reproduce these photographs. I am also indebted to the Wellcome Library of the History of Medicine (London) for making my researches into the history of psychiatric illustration possible through their rich holdings. The Royal Society (London) has graciously allowed publication of Diamond's hitherto unpublished paper on the physiognomy of insanity. The staff of the Olin Library at Cornell has also been of great help in documenting Diamond's career. My special thanks goes to Marianne Horney-Eckardt, M.D., who was able to judge the aesthetic as well as historical merits of Diamond's work.

S.L.G.

Ithaca, New York
June, 1976

CONTENTS

INTRODUCTION

Patients have been depicted throughout the earlier history of medical illustrations primarily in a nonpathognomonic manner. We see them as the recipients of medical action — wounds are being bound, dislocations are reduced, and finally (and unhappily) the patient's dead body is being dissected. This does not mean that the physician is disinterested in the appearance of his patient. Quite to the contrary, for in the patient's look and demeanor lie clues for understanding the nature of his illness and the expected outcome. When Hippocrates wrote about the latter in discussing prognosis, he gave us descriptions that are vividly meaningful to this date.

It is to the great masters of art, however, that we owe an eternal debt for their early representation of emotionally distressed human beings. Many examples of their work could be cited, but one of the most famous of the Renaissance is the portrait of a melancholic woman by Albrecht Dürer. The beautiful drawings and paintings of artists such as Dürer are informative, but did not have an explicit medical purpose.

Jumping rapidly over the centuries to the beginning of the nineteenth, it becomes evident that painting and psychiatry are now moving closer together in the striking work of the short-lived Géricault. His paintings often contain a fervid and moving quality which has been compared to those of Van Gogh. He painted a series of ten portraits of mental patients for his friend, Dr. Étienne-Jean Georget, of which five appear to be lost. Tradition has it that these portraits were planned for a book being written by Georget, who was a brilliant student of Pinel and Esquirol in the growing school of French psychiatry. Recent evidence indicates that Géricault painted his insane fellow patients while he himself was institutionalized under the care of Dr. Georget.

The history of the medical use of portraits has yet to be written. Who was the first to propose it is as yet unknown, but Benjamin Rush in a letter written in 1802 suggested that Gilbert Stuart undertake such a task, stating, "Thirty years ago I communicated to Mr. [Charles Willson] Peale a wish to see a gallery of portraits of sick people laboring under such diseases as show themselves in features and countenance. They are chiefly madness, melancholy, fatuity, consumption, dropsy, jaundice, leprosy, gutta rosea, stone, cancer, colic, dysentery, smallpox, measles, scarlet fever, and plagues of all kinds." Rush continues, "By means of a gallery of portraits such as I have hinted at, the study of medicine might be much aided, and benevolent sympathies be excited in persons who from education, situation, or too much sensibility are precluded from seeing the originals in sick rooms or hospitals."[1] Rush wished to increase human concern for suffering, but recognized that the subject should be presented in a gentle fashion so as not to overwhelm or antagonize the viewer.

In the same decade that Géricault was producing his powerful portrayals, a physician in Great Britain was pioneering the teaching of psychiatry by presenting a series of public lectures. Alexander Morison prepared his *Outlines of Lectures on Mental Diseases* for publication in 1825, and when he rewrote it towards the end of the decade, he discussed, among other topics, the physiognomy of insanity and included several plates. Physiognomy, or the study of human character through facial configuration, had a long history, and received a great impetus in the eighteenth century through the writings of a Swiss theologian and poet, Johann Kasper Lavater. His books were widely translated and reprinted, and aroused general public interest in paying attention to facial characteristics. Phrenology was another movement during this period that furthered this interest. Started in the 1790's by Franz Joseph Gall and propagated throughout the Anglo-American countries by his disciple, Johann Gasper Spurzheim, the phrenologists measured and felt the configurations of heads to determine mental faculties and character traits and illustrated their publications with their findings.

Morison's textbook with its fine engravings was just the harbinger of future trends which would be seen in his subsequent book, *The Physiognomy of Mental Diseases*, which was published in 1838. It contains over one hundred plates of psychiatric patients accompanied with brief case descriptions. Many of the expressions are most recognizable to the modern clinician. Representations of patients during the acute phase of their illness and again after recovery add to the educational value of the pictures. In the same year in France, J.E.D. Esquirol, the famous student of Philippe Pinel and the acknowledged leader of French psychiatry, had issued his massive textbook (*Of Mental Diseases*) which was accompanied by a few striking psychiatric illustrations. Esquirol actually had shared his collections of busts and drawings with Morison when the first illustrated *Outlines* was issued. It was Morison's book, however, that initiated a style of correlating in some depth a person's appearance and his psychopathology — a style that reached a new peak after 1885 from the work of Jean Martin Charcot and Paul Richer in Pinel's old service at the Salpêtrière. Charcot and Richer researched the correlation between art and psychopathology in their *Les Démoniaques dans L'Art* (1887). They followed this work with their serial *Nouvelle Iconographie de la Salpêtrière* (1888–1918), a massive undertaking correlating appearances (signs in medical terminology) with various pathological states (symptoms and diagnosis).

Sander Gilman's researches, therefore, are in the midst of this tradition; through his enterprising efforts he has located a series of marvelous photographs of psychiatric patients taken by a pioneer medical photographer, Dr. Hugh W. Diamond. Fortunately, they had been used by John Conolly, considered by many to be the leading British psychiatrist of the mid-century, in preparing a series of lectures, which included clinical information on many of the patients. Although most of the engravings have been drawn with remarkable fidelity, there is one that should be noted where editorial treatment has brought about a significant change (see plates 1 and 2). It is a photograph of a young woman with religious melancholia and shows her looking firmly at the viewer. In the engraving, her eyes are cast down, making her appear both withdrawn and more depressed. Note also that some books have been placed between her hand and the table; by implication they must be religious tracts that overly concern her.

Until now, these photographs have been known only through the sketches made from them. Professor Gilman has performed a great service in locating them and by giving us their history. I do not know when the first psychiatric photographs appear in a book. Certainly *The Mind Unveiled* (1858) with its photographs of mentally retarded children is an early one of its genre. We shall all look forward to Professor Gilman's further investigations of historical psychiatric illustrations for the answer to many questions.

ERIC T. CARLSON, M.D.
Clinical Professor of Psychiatry
Director, Section on the History
of Psychiatry and the Behavioral Sciences,
New York Hospital-Cornell Medical Center

1. L. H. Butterfield, ed. *Letters of Benjamin Rush* (Philadelphia: American Philosophical Society, 1951.) p. 852.

The Face of Madness

HUGH W. DIAMOND

AND

Psychiatric Photography

BY SANDER L. GILMAN, PH.D.
Chairman, Department of German Literature
Cornell University

Photography is so essentially the Art of Truth—and the representative of Truth in Art—that it would seem to be the essential means of reproducing all forms and structures of which science seeks for delineation . . . . We were therefore surprised in passing through the rooms of the Photographic Society lately, to find so few photographs which had any bearing upon surgery, medicine, and the allied sciences. It is much to be regretted that the great resources of the Photographic Art—seen here in a hundred beautiful forms—have not yet been more fully applied to the purposes of our art.[1]

This complaint graced the pages of the January, 1859 issue of the British medical journal, *Lancet*. Unknown to the author of these sentiments, but fully within his conception of photography, many early amateur photographers had already turned their hobby towards the interests of science, especially the medical arts. Photography, in the England of 1859 no more than twenty years old, was held to be the ultimate form of realistic portrayal. Thus a new type of empirical scientific proof was seen to be possible, as photographers turned their cameras toward recording scientific data. In the late 1830's the Rev. J. B. Reade recorded the image seen through a microscope on a photographic plate and the art of photomicroscopy was born.[2] At the same time, the camera also became a diagnostic tool. One early experiment attempted to record breath patterns in order to determine pathologies of the lung.[3] Nevertheless, these early decades of medical photography were marked by the absence of any systematic use of the photograph in medical procedures.[4] It was in psychiatry, an area which on the first glance would seem singularly unfruitful for the use of the camera, that the first systematic theory and practice of clinical photography were undertaken. The founder of clinical photography was one of the Rev. J. B. Reade's prime disciples, Hugh Welch Diamond, who earned the title of "the father of psychiatric photography."[5]

Diamond was born in 1809 to a middle-class provincial family in Kent. His father had been a surgeon in the service of the East India Company, who, upon his return to England, was elected High Bailiff of Henley-in-Arden (Warwick). Educated at Norwich Grammar School, Diamond studied medicine at the Royal College of Surgeons beginning in 1824. In 1828 he became a student at St. Bartholomew's Hospital (St. Bart's) and soon thereafter opened a private practice in the highly respectable area around Soho Square. During the cholera epidemic of 1832 Diamond played a major role in aiding the ill of this section of London. In 1834 he became a Fellow of the Royal College of Surgeons.

During the 1840's Diamond's interests altered and he became more and more interested in the newly reformed treatment of the insane. The Professor of Medicine at the University of London, John Conolly, had published his initial study of the use of "non-restraint" in 1830, importing Philippe Pinel's reforms of the French asylum into England.[6] However, Diamond undertook his psychiatric studies not at Hanwell Asylum with Conolly but at Bethlem Hospital (Bedlam) under Sir George Tuthill, an advocate of more stringent means of treatment. In 1848 Diamond was elected the resident superintendent of the Female Department of the Surrey County Lunatic Asylum, where he remained until 1858.

The period from 1848 to 1858 was central to Diamond's involvement with clinical psychiatry and photography. In 1839 W. H. Fox Talbot had developed the calotype process which fixed images as negatives, replacing the cumbersome direct method of the daguerreotype.[7] Diamond was extremely influential in disseminating information about this process and other innovations in photography. In the pages of the antiquarian periodical *Notes and Queries* between 1852 and 1854 Diamond published more than a dozen essays and notes on photography, the most important being the republication of a paper read to the Photographic Society in November, 1853 on "The Simplicity of the Calotype Process." This was the first major exposé of the calotype process for amateur photographers, who had been led to believe that this process was much too complicated for their use. With the greater simplicity of the calotype proven, the cheap, easily duplicative photograph became a reality and the craze for the "cartes-de-viste" began. Easily reproducible photographs also had an important implication for medical photography.

Diamond's work in the area of the popularization of photography did not go unrecognized. In 1853 a group of "amateurs of Photography in the city of Norwich" wrote to the editor of *Notes and Queries* their "grateful thanks for the frankness and liberality with which he [Diamond] has published the valuable results of his experiments. . . . We have all profited largely by Dr. Diamond's instructions, and beg to express our conviction that he is entitled to the gratitude of every lover of the Art."[8] A more tangible sign of photography's debt to Diamond came in 1854 when a group of amateurs, among them the physicist Michael Faraday, presented Diamond with a purse of three hundred pounds and a scroll which read: "The improvements effected by Dr. Diamond have been the result of numerous and costly experiments carried on in the true spirit of scientific inquiry, and explained in the most frank and liberal manner, without the slightest reservation or endeavour to obtain from them any private or personal advantage."[9]

Diamond's importance in the history of early English photography was not limited to his technical innovations. He applied the art of photography both to his other hobbies, such as archaeology, and to his profession.[10] In 1852 he presented a series on "the types of insanity" recorded in photographs to a London audience.[11] These portraits were the first systematic use of photography in the history of psychiatry. Standing in the physiognomic tradition of J.E.D. Esquirol, who had more than two hundred patients sketched at Salpêtrière, and Sir Alexander Morison (Diamond's predecessor at the Surrey Asylum), whose major atlas of *The Physiognomy of Mental Diseases* appeared in 1838, Diamond attempted to record the appearance of the insane for clinical use. In 1856 he presented a paper before the Royal Society on his theories of the use of photography in the practice of psychiatry. This paper, which is published here in its entirety for the first time, argued that photography can have three important functions in the treatment of the mentally ill.[12] It can record the appearance of the mentally ill for study (ascribing to the theories of the physiognomy of insanity accepted at that period); it can be used in the treatment of the mentally ill through the presentation of an accurate self-image; and it can record the visages of patients to facilitate identification for later re-admission and treatment.

Diamond's paper was a breakthrough in the development of psychiatric illustration. In 1806 Sir Charles Bell had argued that when one portrayed the insane "it is with a moral aim, to show the consequence of vice and the indulgence of passion."[13] Some years later Esquirol argued that "one can conclude that the study of the physiognomy of the insane is not an object of idle curiosity. Such a study can aid in unraveling the character of the ideas and the emotions which occur during the delirium of such an illness."[14] Esquirol's views were rooted in the new empiricism of the French psychiatric school founded by Pinel, while Bell's comment continued the eighteenth century tradition of the portrayal of madness seen in Hogarth's *The Rake's Progress*. In altering the understanding of the role of the portrayal of the insane and in accepting the portrait as empirical proof of the psychiatric symptomatology, Diamond stood in a major new tradition of the physiognomy of insanity.

In accepting the contemporary view of the photograph as the most realistic presentation possible, Diamond fell into a different error than the earlier portraitists of the insane. The portraits, while readily identifiable within the tradition of psychiatric physiognomy as illustrations of Pinel's categorizations of the insane, were also pre-figured in two recognizable sets of visual models. Esquirol's own illustrations, published first as crude line drawings, in the *Dictionnaire des sciences médicales,* and then as much more detailed engravings accompanying his collected papers in 1838, present many of the same images found in many of Diamond's photographs. These are not inherent in the nature of the illness but rather stem from the posing of the patient, the concentration of the face, and the absence of background. Parallel to this influence are echoes of the contemporary photographic portrait, so well known from the contemporary works of Julia Margaret Cameron and Lewis Carroll. Diamond's photographs give the illusion of reality through the use of existing models. It is this aspect of Diamond's photographs which provides an aesthetic structure. For, while the subject matter is of medical interest, the photographs themselves possess an aesthetic importance through the skillful manipulation of the format to obtain the greatest effect on the observer.

In addition to the use of the photograph as a diagnostic tool in the evaluation of the physiognomy of insanity, Diamond used his photographs in the treatment of the inmates at the Surrey Asylum. In freezing the features of the inmates, the camera was able to present an indelible image of the patient for the patient's own study. These self-images had an effect on some of the inmates, if just because of their novelty. In response to the report of Diamond's paper before the Royal Society, T. N. Brushfield, Superintendent of the Chester County Lunatic Asylum, wrote:

I have not had an opportunity of reading or knowing the contents of Dr. Diamond's paper [on] photography as applied in the treatment, etc. of lunacy, beyond the ordinary newspaper article; but I have found, notwithstanding my imperfect attempts, that patients are very much gratified at seeing their own portraits, and more particularly when associated with a number of others on a large sheet of Bristol board, framed, and hung up as an ordinary picture in the ward. In our worst female ward I have had a positive (on glass) framed and hung up for nearly eighteen months, and it has never yet been touched by any of the patients, although nearly all know whom it represents. Last week a patient, who was formerly one of our most violent cases, begged for a portrait of herself, that she might send to her son, who was in Ireland, to show how much better she was.

In the case of *criminal* lunatics, it is frequently of great importance that a portrait should be obtained, as many of them being originally of criminal disposition and education, if they do escape from the asylum are doubly dangerous to the community at large, and they may frequently be traced by sending their photographs to the police authorities (into whose hands they are very likely to fall) from some act of depredation they are likely to commit; the photographs would thus cause them to be identified, and secure their safe return to the asylum.[15]

The photograph could function as a tool for the treatment of the insane only as long as it remained a novelty.

The use of photographs in medical record keeping, as suggested by Diamond, is now commonplace. While it is not known whether Diamond used his photographs to document the records of his own patients, the idea of the photograph as a record-keeping device was in the air during the early 1850's. From 1851 to 1854 Philip Henry Delamotte recorded the building of the Crystal Palace through photographs. In institutional record keeping, however, the photograph was little known outside of Diamond's suggestion. It became common only during the 1870's when the inmates of the orphan asylums run by Dr. Thomas John Barnardo were photographed to record their altered physical development in their new environment.

With the introduction of the photograph into psychiatry an ethical question was raised: Should one photograph the patients with or without their acquiescence? In the plates provided by Esquirol only one patient was specifically cited as having been willing to have her portrait drawn. Her willingness sprang, however, from her dementia, for she believed herself to be possessed and wanted her portrait presented to the Archbishop for his blessing. Of a photograph taken by Sir William Charles Hood at Bethlem Asylum in the early 1880's there is a more detailed description of the patient's reaction:

After being several weeks at Bethlem, it became practicable to take her portrait; and she was very willing to have it done. In fact, the taking of portraits has become one of the pleasures of which the patients cheerfully partake in our lunatic asylums; and helps, in combination with the various other alleviations studied by humane superintendents, to diversify and cheer the days passed in necessary seclusion from the busier, but scarcely happier world, without. One incidental effect of these artistical amusements is to draw the attention of the patients themselves to their own costume, and sometimes also to their general appearance, as to face and figure; and this direction of their notice may lead to salutary results. In the case in question, the patient made some objection to her own dress, which she evidently thought not very becoming; and she at length made it a condition of her sitting quiet that she should be represented with a book in her hand. The book, indeed, was held upside down; but it did quite as well. Her sense of propriety was gratified, and her face shows that she required no printed page to suggest thoughts to her yet busy mind.[16]

Here the photograph is taken for use in treatment. Whether Diamond obtained permission to photograph his public patients at the Surrey Asylum is unknown. But once he left the Surrey Asylum in 1858 and opened a private asylum in Twickenham House, Middlesex, which he operated until his death on June 21, 1886, he no longer photographed his patients.

During the 1860's Diamond was extremely active in the official affairs of the Photographic Society. He edited its journal from 1859 to 1869, served as its secretary for this period and later as one of its vice-presidents. In 1867 he served on the board of jurors for photography during the Paris Exhibition and in that same year was awarded the medal for excellence of the Photographic Society.

The outgrowth of Diamond's work on the photography of the insane came in 1858 when his photographs of 1852 inspired a major series of essays by John Conolly on "The Physiognomy of Insanity." Here the importance of the photograph as opposed to other forms of illustration can be noted, for even contemporaries noted the marked difference between the original photographs and the lithographs based upon them.

> The late Dr. Conolly, the highest authority on this subject, not only studied attentively numbers of photographs of different forms of insanity brought under his notice, but actually wrote a valuable series of papers in which the varieties of insanity were described by reference to photographs. These were taken by Dr. Diamond from cases then under his care, and are comprised in the collection now laid on the table for your inspection. I have also placed a work containing a lithograph of one of these cases. It is entirely destitute of all those minute points of expression which alone could give any value to such an illustration. But it was the best thing of its kind; and comparison of it with the photograph by Dr. Diamond of the same case will indicate, better than words can tell, the great intrinsic value of photography in thus reproducing minute characteristics of expression.[17]

Most evident in the absence of close detail and in the alteration and reinterpretation of the visage of the patient, the engraving of the photograph altered the value of the illustration but did not destroy it. For an engraved photograph was still a more accurate symptomatological portrayal than an interpretive sketch.

Conolly viewed his essays as a continuation of the work of Esquirol and Morison. However, he viewed his essays as having empirically greater value since they were based on photographs rather than mere drawings:

The modern artist and the photographer are enabled to represent true pictures of what is effected by mental malady, and to facilitate the knowledge of its association with bodily ailment or disturbance, capable of relief.[18]

The fallacy that the photograph presented an objective portrayal of the mentally ill is central to Conolly's understanding of this method. Conolly's essays, while substantially more extensive than Diamond's paper, are therefore of less value. They do not supply the new approach suggested by Diamond and stand clearly in the general tradition of physiognomy begun by Johann Kaspar Lavater in the late eighteenth century. They do, however, supply a series of the missing case studies for some of Diamond's photographs.

Hugh Welch Diamond's theory and practice of psychiatric photography were without parallel in his time, but did not remain without echo. In his paper to the Royal Society, Diamond quoted a letter to him from Ernst Lacan, one of the most active members of the Parisian Photographic Society. In 1856, as part of the celebration of the end of the Crimean War, a photographic exposition was held in Paris. As part of this exhibition Lacan wrote the first general history of photography. In one chapter Lacan mused as to the possible further applications of photography and described his contact with Hugh Diamond and his photographs:

I have before me a collection of fourteen portraits of women of various ages. Some are smiling, others seem to be dreaming. All have something strange in their physiognomy: that is what one sees at first glance. If one ponders them for a longer period of time, one grows sad against one's will. All these faces have an unusual expression which causes pain in the observer. A single word of explanation suffices these are portraits of the insane. These photographs are part of the masterly work of Dr. Diamond, who practices at the Surrey County Asylum near London. In the interest of his art, and to serve the study of mental diseases, Dr. Diamond, one of the most skillful amateur photographers, has had the courage to reproduce the features of the unfortunate women placed under his care. It is with a painful interest that one follows in these portraits, taken at various times, the stages of the disease. One of these unfortunate women, stricken with puerperal insanity, is portrayed four times [Plate 14]. First, on her admission to the institution: she is calm, and yet, her insanity is evident. Her contracted features, deformed through suffering, her straight hair, bristled and tangled, indicate

12   THE FACE OF MADNESS

everything. Another print represents her during an attack. She is laughing, but what a laugh. . . . Here she is convalescing. Her face recovers a more peaceful appearance, the features regain their position and soften. Finally she is restored to health. If one takes the final portrait and compares it to the initial one, one will be able to judge the perturbations which insanity produces in the human physiognomy. These four prints speak more than a whole book. Others represent various kinds of mental illness: nymphomania, incurable insanity, insanity accompanied by epilepsy, suicidal monomania. The last one, the most unusual one perhaps, is the portrait of an unfortunate old woman who has been in a complete state of catalepsy for five months. Dr. Diamond has portrayed her seated in an armchair with her legs stretched, her head erect, her eyes shut convulsively. It is the rigidity and immobility of death.

If Dr. Diamond's example is followed, as we hope it will be, how many such valuable collections can be formed, how many scientific treasures will be added to those already in our museums and medical schools.[19]

Lacan's opinion was widely discussed. Within the next year the first documented use of clinical photography in the recording of the physiognomy of the insane to illustrate a medical text appeared in the atlas to B. A. Morel's *Traité des dégénérescences physiques, intellectuelles et morales de l'espèce humaine et des causes que produisent ces variétés maladises.*[20] The tenth plate in this atlas contains a lithograph of two cretins based on a photograph taken by Baillarger at Salpêtrière. Thus, as early as 1857 the photograph began to play a major role in psychiatric illustration under the influence of Hugh W. Diamond's early experiments.

NOTES

1. *Lancet,* January 22, 1859, p. 89.

2. R. D. Wood, "J. B. Reade's early photographic experiments: Recent and further evidence in the legend," *British Journal of Photography* 119 (1972), 643–647.

3. The early experiments in the application of photography to medicine are discussed in the first survey of this question, H. G. Wright, "On the medical uses of photography," *The Photographic Journal* 9 (1867), 202–204.

4. The question of the evolution of clinical photography has been little studied; see H. S. Dommasch, "The development of medical photography," *Journal of the Biological Photographic Association* 33 (1965), 169–170; Norman Kiell, ed., *Psychiatry and Psychology in the Visual Arts and Aesthetics* (Madison and Milwaukee: University of Wisconsin Press, 1965); Alison Gernsheim, "Medical photography in the nineteenth century," *Medical and Biological Illustration* 11 (1961), 85–92; "Victorian clinical photography," *Medical and Biological Illustration* 9 (1959), 70–77.

5. Little is known of Diamond's life except for the detailed obituary in *The Athenaeum* (1886), 17–18 and the standard reference books of the period, such as *The Medical Directory for 1886* (London: J & A Churchill, 1886), 526. The standard biographic essays on Diamond, such as that in the *Dictionary of National Biography*, V, 906, are based on these sources. The most recent mention of Diamond's psychiatric work is in Cecil Beaton and Gail Buckland, *The Magic Image: The Genius of Photography from 1839 to the Present Day* (London: Weidenfeld and Nicolson, 1975), p. 48. The absence of all primary material was determined as early as 1926 by Charles Oakum in his research on J. B. Reade; see letters from Oakum to R. Hugh Clark, Diamond's grandson, dated April 13, 1926 and April 23, 1926 in the possession of the Medical Society of London.

6. The general histories of psychiatry fail to mention Diamond. Only Richard Hunter and Ida Macalpine, eds., *Three Hundred Years of Psychiatry: A History Presented in Selected English Texts* (London: Oxford University Press, 1963), p. 1033 refer to him. Valuable in general is the documentation by Vieda Skultans, ed., *Madness and Morals: Ideas on Insanity in the Nineteenth Century* (London: Routledge and Kegan Paul, 1975), especially pp. 71–98.

7. For a general survey of the history of photography with some references to Diamond's role in the Photographic Society see Helmut Gernsheim, *The History of Photography from the Camera Obscura to the Beginning of the Modern Era* (London: Thames and Hudson, 1969). Diamond's relationship to early British photographers is documented in the diaries of Lewis Carroll, who visited him on January 18, 1856. [Roger Lancelyn Green, ed., *The Diaries of Lewis Carroll* (London: Cassell, 1953), I, 74.]

8. *Notes and Queries* 7 (1853), 93. Among Diamond's essays on photography were the following: From *Notes and Queries* 6 (1852): "On French collodion," 470; "On photography applied to the microscope," 562; 7 (1853), "On the originator of the collodion process," 92; "On collodion pictures," 582; "Processes upon paper," 20–23; 8 (1853), "On the collodion process," 133; "On the calotype process," 548, 596; "Process for printing on allumenised paper," 324–26; "On the simplicity of the calotype process," 596–600; 10 (1854) "On iodizing paper," 192; 11 (1855) "On bromo-iodide of silver," 130; "How to deepen a positive collodion picture into a good printing negative," 371; "On the fading of positives," 110; N.S. 1 (1856), "The application of photography to the copying of ancient documents, prints, pictures, coins, etc.," 160. From *The Photographic Journal* 1 (1854), "On the simplicity of the calotype process," 129–132; 2 (1856), "On amber varnish," 11; 8 (1864), "On a singular and interesting instance of polychrome in a photograph," 21; "On protection to photographs in the Copyright Bill," 23–24; "Processing several colours," 41.

9. Quoted in *The Athenaeum* obituary, *op. cit.*, 17.

10. "The application of photography to archaeology," *Notes and Queries* 6 (1852), 276–8, 295–6, 319–20, 371–3.

11. The dating of Diamond's first exhibition of his clinical portraits is taken from the posthumous essay by H. G. Wright, "Medico-photography," *The Photographic Journal* 14 (1869), 133. The location of this exhibition is questionable. It was most probably at the Royal Medico-Chirurgical Society (later the Royal Society for Medicine). Though there is an oblique reference in the 1852 volume of *Notes and Queries* that some of Diamond's "specimens were exhibited at Lord Rosse's soirées during last season" (193), these can hardly have been Diamond's clinical photographs.

12. The entire text of this paper is published in this volume. A summary of this paper appeared in the *Saturday Review* 2 (1856), 81 and was reprinted in *The Photographic Journal* 3 (1856), 88–89. The manuscript of this paper, in Diamond's hand, is to be found in the archives of the Royal Society, London, A.P. 38.22.

13. Sir Charles Bell, *The Anatomy and Philosophy of Expression as Connected with the Fine Arts* (London: C. Bell, 1883), p. 162. See also Ronald Paulson, *Hogarth's Graphic Works* (New Haven: Yale University Press, 1965) I, 169–70.

14. *Des Maladies Mentales, considérées sous les rapports médical, hygiénique et médico-légal* (Paris: J. B. Baillière, 1838), II, 167; translation by the author. See also George Rosen, "The Philosophy of Ideology and the Emergence of Modern Medicine in France," *Bulletin of the History of Medicine* 20 (1946), 329–339.

15. *The Photographic Journal* 3 (1857), 289.

16. John Conolly, "The Physiognomy of Insanity: No. 9, Religious Mania," *The Medical Times and Gazette* N.S. 16 (1858), 83. Conolly's papers "On the Physiognomy of Insanity" ran as follows in *The Medical Times and Gazette*: N.S. 16 (1858) No. 1, "Religious Melancholy," 2–4; No. 2, "Suicidal Melancholy," 56–58; No. 3, "General Melancholia," 134–136; No. 4, "Melancholia passing on to Mania," 238–241; No. 5, "Mania and Convalescence," 314–316; No. 6, "Chronic Mania and Melancholy," 397–398; No. 7, "Senile Dementia," 498–500; No. 8, "Puerperal Mania," 623–624; N.S. 17 (1858) No. 9, "Religious Mania," 81–83; No. 10, "Religious Mania-Convalescence," 210–212; No. 11, "Religious Melancholia," 367–369; No. 12, "Insanity supervening on Habits of Intemperance," 651–653; N.S. 18 (1859) No. 13, "Illustrations of the Old Methods of Treatment," 183–186.

17. Wright, "On the medical uses of photography," *op. cit.*, p. 204. Compare the views of the anonymous author of "The first principle of physiognomy," *Cornhill Magazine* 4 (1861), 570:

It is equally true that with such portraits and engravings of portraits as we have had, it has been utterly impossible to get beyond the nebulous science of a Lavater. We required the photograph. Certainly it looks a hard thing to say that the great portrait-painters are not to be trusted. Is it to be supposed that these masters did not know their business, and have failed to give us correct likenesses of the persons who sat to them? It must be remembered that to give a general likeness is one of the easiest strokes of art. With half-a-dozen lines the image is complete, as anyone may see in the million wood-engravings of the day; while at the same time it would be difficult to gather from these rough sketches, where two dots go for the eyes and a scratch for the mouth, what is the precise anatomy of any one feature. So while we can accept as in the main truthful the portraits that have come down to us, it is impossible to place perfect reliance on any particular lineament.

18. John Conolly, "The Physiognomy of Insanity: No. 3, General Melancholia," 136. Not all of the lithographs accompanying Conolly's essays are taken from photographs by Diamond. At least two are from photographs supplied by William Charles Hood from Bethlem Hospital.

19. Ernst Lacan, *Esquisses photographiques à propos de l'exposition universelle et de la guerre d'orient* (Paris: A. Gaudin, 1856), pp. 40–1; translation by the author.

20. *Atlas de XII. Planches* (Paris: J. B. Baillière, 1857).

ON THE

Application of Photography

TO THE

Physiognomic and Mental

Phenomena of Insanity

BY HUGH W. DIAMOND

Read before the Royal Society, May 22, 1856.

It would never be expected, a priori, that a new science could arrive at any thing like maturity in the space of fifty years, yet with respect to Photography we witness the gratifying fact that the early labours of Wedgwood, Davy, and Young, at the commencement of the present century, have been so zealously followed up, that the fundamental difficulties in the theory of this new science have been overcome and its practical rules very generally established — That I have been a fellow worker with those who have obtained these valuable results will always be a source of the highest pleasure, and I think I shall not be looked upon as presenting a premature offering if I venture to lay before the Royal Society a short account of the peculiar application of Photography which my position in the Surrey Asylum has enabled me to make.

The investigation of the phenomena of Insanity can never be looked upon as a subject of but little interest in a country which has provided so largely for the treatment of Mental derangement — The Metaphysician and Moralist, the Physician and Physiologist will approach such an inquiry with their peculiar views, definitions and classifications — The Photographer, on the other hand, needs in many cases no aid from any language of his own, but prefers rather to listen, with the picture before him, to the silent but telling language of nature — It is unnecessary for him to use the vague terms which denote a difference in the degree of mental suffering, as for instance, distress, sorrow, deep sorrow, grief, melancholy, anguish, despair; the picture speaks for itself with the most marked pression and indicates the exact point which has been reached in the scale of unhappiness between the first sensation and its utmost height — similarly the modification of fear, and of the more painful passions, anger and rage, jealousy and envy, (the frequent concomitants of insanity) being shown from the life by the Pho-

tographer, arrest the attention of the thoughtful observer more power-
fully than any laboured description. — What words can adequately
describe either the peculiar character of the palsy which accompanies
sudden terror when without hope, or the face glowing with heat under
the excitement of burning anger, or the features shrunk and the skin
constricted and ghastly under the influence of pale rage? — Yet the
Photographer secures with unerring accuracy the external phenomena
of each passion, as the really certain indication of internal derangement, and exhibits to the eye the well known sympathy which exists
between the diseased brain and the organs and features of the body —

An Asylum on a large scale supplies instances of delirium with raving fury and spitefulness, or delirium accompanied with an appearance
of gaiety and pleasure in some cases, and with constant dejection and
despondency in others, or imbecility of all the faculties, with a stupid
look and general weakness, and the Photographer catches in a moment
the permanent cloud, or the passing storm or sunshine of the soul, and
thus enables the metaphysician to witness and trace out the connexion
between the visible and the invisible in one important branch of his
researches into the Philosophy of the human mind.

M. Esquirol has described in a striking and accurate manner the
aspect of the countenance peculiar to that stage of dementia which is
characterized by confirmed incoherence, a chronic mania (of which I
exhibit two illustrative portraits) but those who never witness this
exhibition of human suffering, either in the original or in the copy
drawn to the life, can hardly imagine this peculiar state of mental
prostration —

Professor Heinroth gives a graphic description of the Phenomena
of raving madness in cases which display the greatest intensity of the
disease — In the first stage we witness the forehead contracted, the
eyebrows drawn up, the hair bristled, and the eye-balls prominent as
if pushed out of their orbits — In the second stage nothing can be compared to the truly satanic expression of the countenance, and the phenomena of the loss of reason in their greatest intensity — and in the
third stage, the violent paroxysms cease, the countenance is pallid and
meagre, and the disease subsides into a permanent fatuity — Photography, as is evident from the portraits which illustrate this paper, con-

firms and extends this description, and that to such a degree as warrants the conclusion that the permanent records thus furnished are at once the most concise and the most comprehensive.

There is another point of view in which the value of portraits of the Insane is peculiarly marked. – viz. in the effect which they produce upon the patients themselves – I have had many opportunities of witnessing this effect – In very many cases they are examined with much pleasure and interest, but more particularly in those which mark the progress and cure of a severe attack of Mental Aberration – I may particularly refer to the four portraits [see Plate 14] which represent different phases of the case of the same young person commencing with that stage of Mania which is marked by the bristled hair, the wrinkled brow, the fixed unquiet eye, and the lips apart as if from painful respiration, but passing, not to a state in which no man could tame her, but happily through less excited stages to the *perfect* cure – In the third portrait the expression is tranquil and accompanied with the smile of sadness instead of the hideous laugh of frenzy – The Hair falls naturally and the forehead alone retains traces, tho' slight ones, of mental agitation. In the fourth there is a perfect calm – The poor maniac is cured. This patient could scarcely believe that her last portrait representing her as clothed and in her right mind, would even have been preceded by anything so fearful; and she will never cease, with these faithful monitors in her hand, to express the most lively feelings of gratitude for a recovery so marked and unexpected – I feel that I shall be supported by the Chaplain to our Asylum if I show a moral truth from these portraits, which, if I apprehend it rightly amounts to this – that religion can win its way to hearts barred against every other influence, that it can soften and conquer dispositions which would else remain intractable and savage; and that hereby in addition to all its other and higher merits, it establishes a title to be considered the great humanizer of Mankind.

It is of course beside my purpose to allude to the value of Photographic Physiognomy in marking the varied Phenomena of sane mental power as exhibited in the different cast of countenance in the Philosopher, the Mathematician, the Poet, etc. but I may observe that the study of Physiognomy is equally necessary when tracing the characteristic features of different mental diseases in their commencement, continuance, and cure. Nor in a sanitary point of view is it unimportant, for many a time the practised eye of the physican may see the storm approaching and by remedial and preventive measures, can greatly subdue its force.

There are cases however in which the most anxious forethought and watchful care are of no avail; and this was the case with the unhappy patient whose small portrait is placed fifth in the frame — It cannot be examined without deep interest and it is thus described by M. Ernest Lacan of Paris —

[One's eyes are captured by the portrait of a woman tormented by suicidal monomania. This woman, of a mature age, must have been quite attractive when in the bloom of youth. Misfortune came, and then illness, but they did not succeed in depriving her features of their beautiful composure. And yet, what sadness, how many complaints, how many disappointments are to be found in those eyes! What anxieties, morbid thoughts and ominous schemes are written on this wrinkled forehead. How many tears, scarcely dried, are on these shrivelled cheeks. How much bitterness and restrained grief, how many swallowed sobs, are in this mouth, whose smile must have been so graceful in the past!

Should not the expression of despair stamped upon this pallid face show a profound revulsion against life and the omnipresence of morbid thoughts, the wide scar this unfortunate person bears on her throat would reveal all. This photograph is a moving drama.]*

After this description, almost prophetic in its terms, it will scarcely excite surprise if I state that this patient, after many cunning but disappointed attempts, eventually carried out her fatal purpose and Photography has recorded the last page in the fearful drama — of this last picture M. Lacan says

[This photograph provides much material for study and reflection. The woman's face, cramped while alive, has recovered its serenity in death. Calmness has come upon these features, so recently convulsively agitated; her half-opened eyes, her almost smiling mouth, seem to express the satisfaction of satiated desire. Is this a final symptom of her illness, or did reason return at the hour of death, giving this unfortunate woman the

*The original passage is in French.

feeling of finally being freed from a life of misery and grief. Only science can answer this. . .]*

As a contrast to this melancholy story I may refer with pleasure to a case in which Photography unquestionably led to the cure.

A.D. aged 20 was admitted under my care in August 1854, having been recently discharged uncured from Bethlem Hospital after a year's residence there — Her delusions consisted in the supposed possession of great wealth, and of an exalted station as a queen. Any occupation was therefore looked upon by her as beneath her dignity. I wished to possess portraits of the several patients who imagined themselves to be Queens and Royal personages, and one of these in a dominant attitude and with a band or "diadem" round the head, stands first in the frame. It was however not without much persuasion that I induced the Queen, A.D., to give me the honour of a sitting — I told her that it was my wish to take portraits of all the Queens under my care, and I will remember the contempt with which she observed "Queens indeed! ! How did they obtain their titles?" — I replied, as she did *They imagined them* — "No!" she said sharply, "I never imagine such foolish delusions, they are to be pitied, but *I* was born a Queen." — Her subsequent amusement in seeing the portraits and her frequent conversation about them was the first decided step in her gradual improvement, and about four months ago she was discharged perfectly cured, and laughed heartily at her former imaginations —

The illustrative portraits to which I have not specially alluded — viz. the example of melancholy, in which even the hands speak the language of melancholy, the type of Epileptic Mania, and some of the smaller portraits, for the most part tell their own tale, with perhaps the exception of the remarkable illustration of catalepsy as exhibited in the patient who is seated in an arm chair with her body erect, the hands raised to the height of the eyes, the arms rigid, and the whole face imprinted with the characters of death — In this position or in any other in which she might be placed she would remain motionless and insensible for hours. — The portraits of the insane are valuable to Superintendents of Asylums for reference in cases of re-admission. It

*The original passage is in French.

is well known that the portraits of those who are congregated in prisons for punishment have often times been of much value in re-capturing some who have escaped, or in proving with little expense, and with certainty a previous conviction; and similarly the portraits of the Insane who are received into Asylums for protection, give to the eye so clear a representation of their case that on their re-admission after temporary absence and cure — I have found the previous portrait of more value in calling to my mind the case and treatment, than any verbal description I may have placed on record.

In conclusion I may observe that Photography gives permanence to these remarkable cases, which are types of classes, and makes them observable not only now but for ever, and it presents also a perfect and faithful record, free altogether from the painful caricaturing which so disfigures almost all the published portraits of the Insane as to render them nearly valueless either for purposes of art or of science.

CASE STUDIES

FROM

The Physiognomy of Insanity

BY JOHN CONOLLY

The Medical Times and Gazette (1858)

WITH

P L A T E S   1–17

The engraving presented to the reader in this number is from a photographic portrait of a young woman labouring under religious melancholy. In this form of melancholy there is no mere worldly despondency, nor thought of common calamities or vulgar ruin; but a deeper horror: a fixed belief, against which all arguments are powerless, and all consolation vain; a belief of having displeased the Great Creator, and of being hopelessly shut out from mercy and from heaven. This portrait, therefore, does not reflect the figure of patients so often recognised in asylums, sitting on benches by the lonely walls, the hands clasped on the bosom, the leaden eye bent on the ground, and the unvarying gloom excluding variety of reflection. It represents an affliction more defined. We discern the outward marks of a mind which, seemingly, after long wandering in the mazes of religious doubt, and struggling with spiritual niceties too perplexing for human solution, is now overshadowed by despair. The high and wide forehead, generally indicative of intelligence and imagination; the slightly bent head, leaning disconsolately on the hand; the absence from that collapsed cheek of every trace of gaiety; the mouth inexpressive of any varied emotion; the deep orbits and the long characteristic eyebrows; all seem painfully to indicate the present mood and general temperament of the patient. The black hair is heedlessly pressed back; the dress, though neat, has a conventual plainness; the sacred emblem worn round the neck is not worn for ornament. The lips are well-formed, and compressed; the angle of the jaw is rather large; the ear seems well-shaped; force of character appears to be thus indicated, as well as a capacity of energetic expression; whilst the womanly figure, the somewhat ample chest and pelvis (less expressed in the engraving than in the photograph) belong to a general constitution out of which, in health and vigour, may have grown up some self-accusing thoughts in an innocent and devout, but passionate heart. For this perverting malady makes even the natural instincts appear sinful; and the suf-

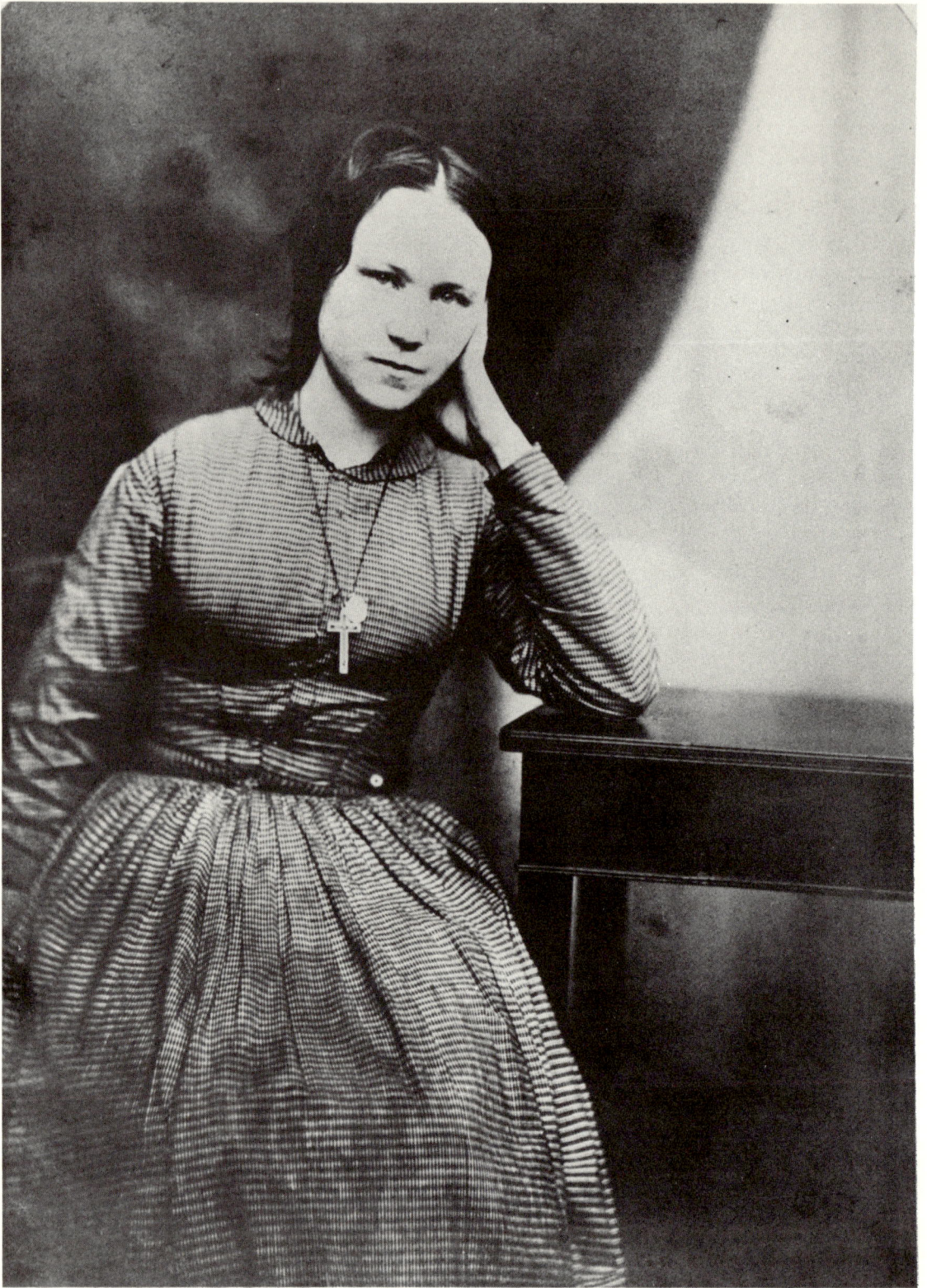

PLATE 1

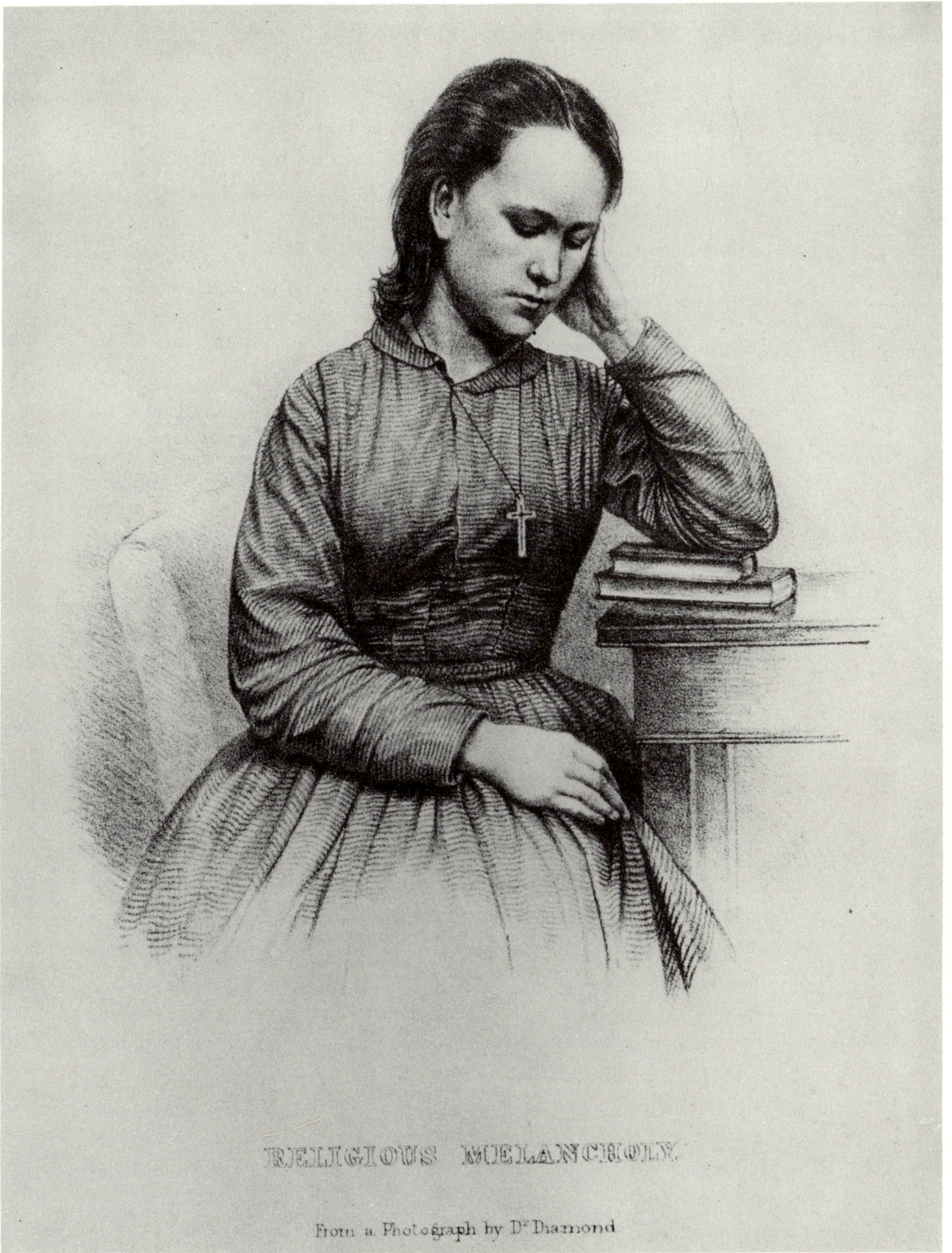

RELIGIOUS MELANCHOLY.

From a Photograph by Dr Diamond

PLATE 2

ferer forgets that God implanted them. But the conflict in the case before us is chiefly intellectual. The meditations of that large brain are not employed on worldly cares, nor even on affections chilled, nor temporal hopes broken. They are engaged in religious scruples, far too perplexing for its power to overcome. In the meantime all the ordinary affections, from which consolation might be derived, are shut out. Soon, perhaps, the scruples themselves will appear crimes. To escape future punishment, bodily mortifications must be endured, severe fasts, or some self-inflicted pain. Under these, the bodily strength, usually impaired in the commencement of the attack, becomes further impaired. The digestion becomes feeble, and even the sparest meals occasion suffering. Emaciation takes place; often proceeding to an extreme degree. The uterine functions (for the subjects of this form of malady are usually women), are suppressed. Paroxysms of excitement may occur, with sudden activity in the prosecution of schemes of vaguest import; but with these futile efforts misgivings become mingled. The thought of suicide, often suggested, becomes fixed; and such varied and ingenious efforts are made to carry it into effect as to demand incessant vigilance. Yet, even in this state there may be days in which the mind is tranquillised, and needle-work is resumed, or the music of happier times is played once more. But these gleams are transient. The mind loses its energy; debility invades every function; pulmonary or mesenteric disease supervenes; the limbs become anasarcous; and the wretched patient is only relieved by death.

The subjects of this kind of affliction are often highly intellectual, and this seems to endow them with greater latitude of terrible delusions, and with an eloquence in describing them that cannot always be listened to without emotion; seconded as it is by an expression of countenance full of real horror, and significant of the state of utter spiritual abandonment and degradation into which the patient asserts herself to be plunged, without hope of relief on earth or pardon in heaven.

The medical treatment of religious melancholy is often of more import than that which enthusiastic and very well-meaning persons are too much inclined to resort to. Remonstrances, and the perusal of sermons, and of the tracts scattered over too many drawing-room tables, and showered with mischievous, although well-intentioned, activity among the poor, — nay, even the exclusive reading of the Bible and Prayer-book, — must often be refrained from or forbidden. There are states of mind in which the medical man must have courage to exclude these as poisons. The mind must be diverted to more common and more varied subjects, and the bodily health must have the most careful consideration.

These observations apply to all religious sects. The subject of this photograph had left the Protestant faith, and become what is commonly called a Roman Catholic. Her education had not been such as to enable her to reason well on either side, and she became merely wavering and unsettled in her belief. Attention to ordinary matters was neglected; she sat in the attitude shown in the engraving for a long time together; she was negligent of her dress, and occasionally destructive of it. Often she cried out that she was a brute, and had no soul to be saved. Now and then she had a desire to see some minister of religion, either Catholic or Protestant; and soon afterward would refuse to see either, declaring that neither could be useful to her. All this seems to be expressed in the photograph. The medal she wears was given to her by a gentleman connected with the Catholic establishment.

It is unnecessary to say that her case was managed in the asylum with the most prudent caution. She was encouraged to more bodily exertion; and her mental perplexities, not being aggravated by reasonings unadapted to her, gradually died away. She soon began to occupy herself, and became useful in the laundry of the establishment. She was strengthened by quinine. The inactivity of the digestive canal, so common, or so constant in cases of melancholia, was counteracted by combining the decoctum aloes compositum with a tonic; and shower-baths, of half a minute's duration, contributed to restore general bodily energy. Such attacks never yield at once. They come on gradually, and depart slowly. After a residence of ten months in the asylum, this patient became well. It is gratifying to know that she remains well, having now left the institution seven months since.

The change presented by the countenance after recovery from severe mental disturbance is generally remarkable, and sometimes even surprising. In case of acute mania it is singularly marked; and in the particular form of religious melancholy the cheerful smile that supplants the dismal and anxious look of the patient is almost magical. In the case now referred to, whatever there was of meditative or intellectual cast in the face during the period of melancholy, was almost wholly lost when the attack went off. The ample forehead, of course, remained, and the deep orbits; but the eyes, when open, were small and inexpressive, and the mouth seemed to have become commonplace. Her whole appearance was, indeed, so simply that of an uneducated Irish girl, that the very neat gown, cloak, and bonnet, in which she was dressed by the kindness of those about her, seemed incongruous and peculiar. A second photograph, taken at that time, possesses, therefore, little interest. In some other instances the metamorphoses effected by malady and recovery may be usefully, and even instructively represented.

PLATES 3 & 4

The portrait accompanying the present paper represents a different variety of melancholia, but one of equal suffering to the patients, who are haunted, not by spiritual doubts, but by bodily fear, and chiefly of some terrible danger impending over themselves or their families; danger menaced by unknown enemies, above, about, or underneath.

It is evidently not the portrait of an educated or refined person, but a woman of the poorer ranks of life, — from which ranks our large crowded county asylums are filled. How people in such ranks contrived to live, and the kind of life they led before being sheltered there, is intimately known to few who attempt to write about them. They are usually even laborious, because want is ever in view. It is not the fear of difficulties and embarrassments which makes them rise early, and causes them to lie down exhausted with fatigue; it is the fear, nay the certainty, of starvation, if they are idle. So the best among them toil on until they rest in the grave; when, and not till when, their weary task is done. And the worst of them, too impatient of this lot, or tempted beyond their strength, deviate from the walks of industry into the side-paths of idleness and gin, of dissipation and sensuality, become instructed in thieving and other short ways to immediate gain, and die in their own manner. It is easy to moralize on these things, and virtuously to condemn; but God alone can judge such matters justly. If a man would try to do so, he must realise to himself an almost unfurnished home, and hungry children, and rent to pay, and scanty and coarse food day after day, and wretched clothing, giving poor protection against the "heat o' the sun" and "the tedious winter rages." He must fancy the state of his mind under the privation of all indulgences and all amusements, and in the utter absence of all comfortable recreation for mind or body. Who is there, more happily placed, who can estimate or even imagine the physiological results of all this combination of misery and privation? Imperfect digestion and

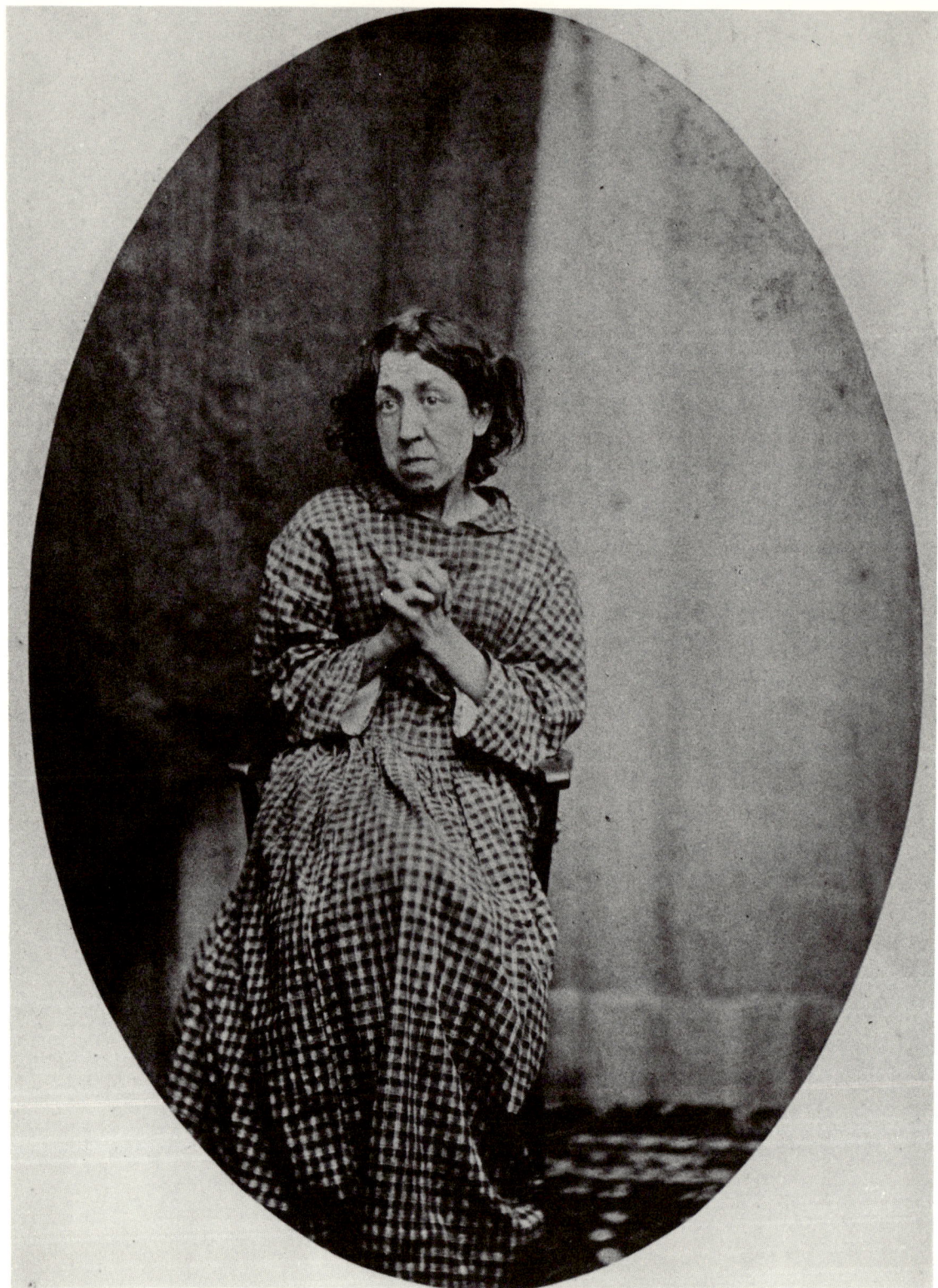

PLATE 3

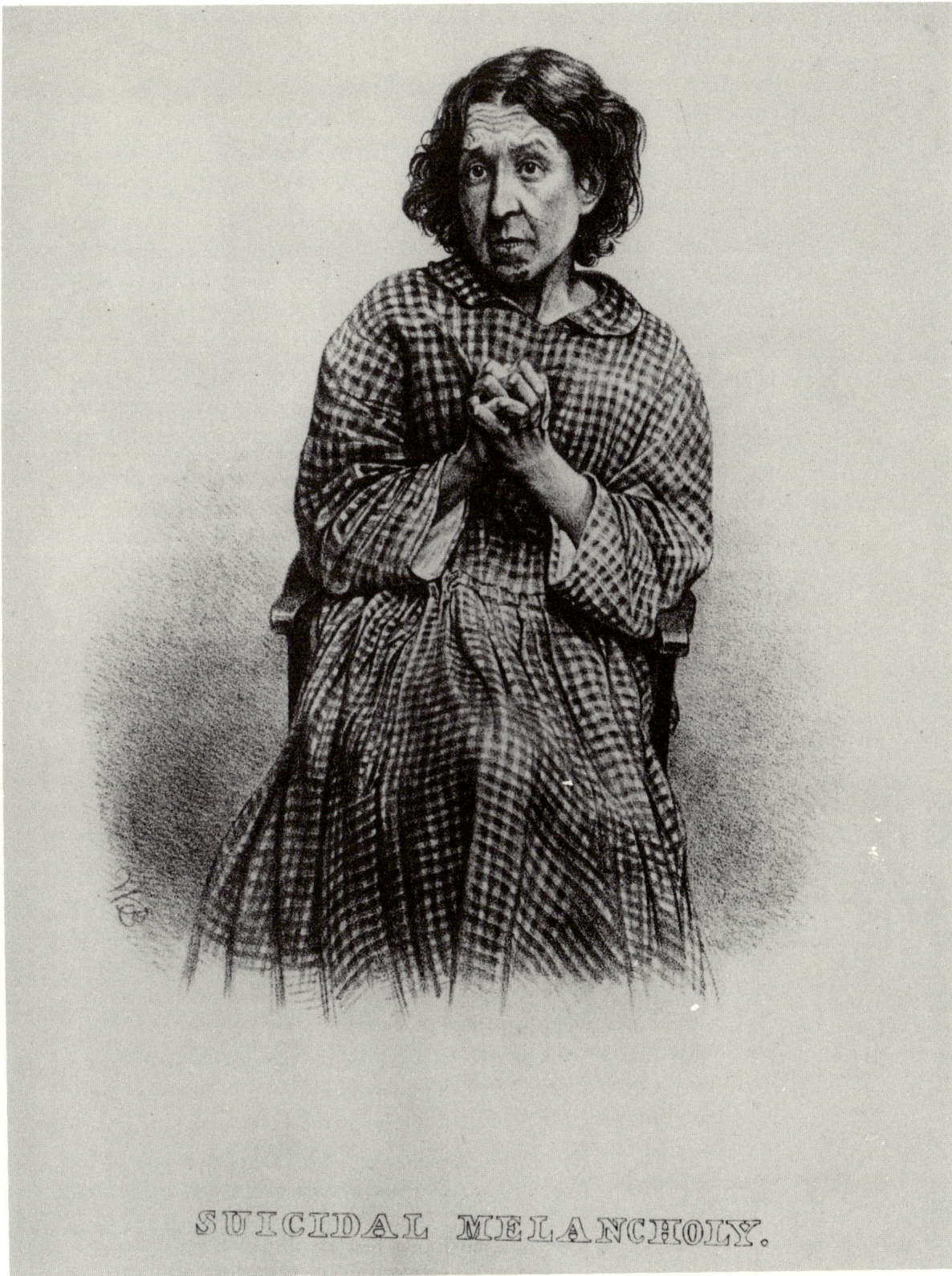

SUICIDAL MELANCHOLY.

PLATE 4

nutrition; the impoverishment of the blood; the consequent deterioration of all the bodily tissues; the lowered character of the grey and white substances of the brain, involving the limitation of the supply of nervous force to all parts of the frame, to those subserving physical offices, and to those of which the integrity is essential to the exercise of the mental and moral faculties; — all these are consequences which may not unreasonably be supposed to ensue to a greater or less extent. But the same causes continue to act in countless families, generation after generation, are transmitted and retransmitted, and their effects accumulated and multiplied; so modifying the general development of the human being that we read even in the face of the bare-footed boy, in the streets of London, his woeful inheritance, and in the features and figure of the grown-up man or woman, in their speech and movement, their wretched physical history. Perhaps we may read something more printed there; the connexion of some, at least, of their faults, or vices, or crimes with the associated impoverishment, if it may be so called, of their higher faculties. We remark the ungainliness of the bodily shape and motion, and the pallor or the unhealthy suffusion of the face, and the ruggedness of the voice and language. With these marks of a degraded type we feel that there can hardly fail to be a corresponding mental limitation. With a total want of instruction there is, in fact, so unobservant a mind that they receive no knowledge from natural objects, and their natural theology is less advanced than that of the poor Indian who sees God in clouds or hears him in the wind. It is unnecessary to go further, now, into these sad particulars. But there is something unreasonable in expecting many excellences to flourish and Christian virtues to find existence in a soil so unprepared. Medical men, and those thoughtful persons, now happily not a few, who are devoting themselves to the advancement of social science, or the real science of living the life befitting so highly endowed a creature as man, do not ignore these painful facts, nor look unheedingly upon them. To physicians who reflect on the cases coming under their care in the wards of our lunatic asylums for the poor, such facts are daily presented as material for serious thought.

In the general appearance of the patient, whose face and figure are copied in the photograph before me, there is something, surely, indicative of at least a few of the points which have been dwelt upon.

At first sight the portrait seems only that of a plain face, almost vulgar. Examined more closely, it becomes affecting. It speaks not of despondency merely, but of some horrible vision that has arisen in the mind. The hands are not only joined, as in ordinary example of profound melancholy, but clasped, almost convulsively, finger within finger, with a muscular energy the expression of which the engraver has most ably caught from the faithful photograph. By this wonderful art the muscles also of the right forearm are depicted as almost in immediate action; and the whole attitude of the patient shows the preponderating muscular strain existing on the same side of the body. The right shoulder is advanced; the right knee is drawn up and pressed on the left. The inclination of the head to the right, the starting muscles on the left side of the neck, the excessive corrugation of the integuments of the forehead, all tell the same story of intense and painful emotion. All this energetic contraction seems to be produced by some fearful feeling. A further perusal of the face tells more than is revealed to a careless glance. The features are unrefined; but the wide and high head indicates intellectual qualities that cultivation might have improved; so as to control, perhaps a now dominating ideality. The copious and dishevelled hair, which we feel sure must be black mingled with grey, is parted with no care, but straggles in sympathy with the tortured brain. Those many and curved wrinkles in the brow are not wrinkles of ordinary trouble. The raised and equally curved eyebrows; the large, melancholy, and uplifted eyes, declare that the sense is fixed on some image of fear, which no other eye can detect; and the intensity of the prevalent emotion is forcibly expressed in all the other parts of the face. The upper eyelids disappear; the lower are strongly depressed; the muscles of the cheeks and the corners of the mouth are drawn down, the lower lip being, as it were, spasmodically acted upon, showing nearly all the front teeth of the lower jaw. The chin has been scratched and scarred by her own finger-nails. The very ears seem starting forward. Everything bespeaks terror. You see that the suffering woman moves not; and that she holds little communion with those about her. Her whole aspect is intensely sorrowful, as well as full of alarm. She is, indeed, abstracted from the common world of sorrow and suffering, but lives in a world of dread alone.

A professed physiognomist, to which title I myself lay no claim, would say that in the face of this poor woman, a certain superiority of character was manifest, although subdued by disease. The long square jaw, the developed chin, the large nose, the compressed and long upper lip, would furnish a text for a pupil of Lavater; and a phrenologist would draw clear conclusions from the configuration of the head. There may be something of fancy, but there is much more of truth in both of these sciences of observation, some acquaintance with which every one desirous to be an accurate observer ought to possess.

The actual history of this patient too well illustrated the miscellaneous remarks which have been offered to the reader. She was born of a mother on whom wretchedness had already done its work; and who was eccentric in mind, and eventually became paralysed. Her sole inheritance was poverty and labour, and a brain disposed to disease. In the portrait she looks old and worn, her real age being only 34. She was industrious, and led a correct life, and for a time managed to earn a living by straw-bonnet making. But this kind of labour is not very profitable, and, in order to ensure food and clothing, and the shelter of a roof, it was necessary for her to work fourteen hours a day. No pleasures, no healthful exercise, were part of her lot. Her mind was of an anxious cast; and she ever felt, no doubt, that the intermission of toil for a day or two would entail difficulty upon her, or the prospect of starvation. What other fears haunted the poor creature we cannot say; but after her mind had quite given way, her often-repeated expressions were, "Oh! don't kill me, dear doctor!" "Don't let any one kill me!" At other times she would say, "I am too wicked to live!" and then she would humbly say that she had not committed any wickedness; but had always been an industrious and good girl. The dread, however, of being murdered grew stronger and stronger. She still worked on, with no salutary variety of any kind, until, with the inconsistency of insanity, she began to think she might escape the danger by destroying her own life. She made many and desperate attempts to do this; attempts only frustrated by the watchfulness of those about her, and by the arrangements of a well-ordered asylum. She would conceal bits of window glass and try to cut her throat; or tear off a strip of sheeting, and throw it quickly over one of the gas-burners in the gallery in order to hang herself. But vigilance saved her again and again from the first danger, and she was preserved from the second by the slight fixing of the burners, made with a prospective regard to such possibilities. The longest experience of the success of these and other attentions to the condition and propensities of the melancholic and suicidal, can yet scarcely make it intelligible how so very large a majority of these cases in asylums are safely managed throughout. If life can be preserved, the wish to die may leave the mind. So long as it remains, so long must the anxious solicitude of the attendants and the Physician continue. And still sometimes, after days and nights of care, a catastrophe may ensue. So fixed does the resolve of self-destruction remain in the poor distracted mind, and so preternatural an ingenuity is exerted in discovering the means of accomplishing it.

JOHN CONOLLY

PLATES 5 & 6

The subject of the illustration accompanying the present paper is one presenting the kind of solemn hopelessness arising out of long and unavailing efforts to keep just above poverty; and out of the diminution of nervous energy which becomes generally perceptible in the working man at his time of life. Probably both circumstances conjoined have brought him to this. He is sixty years old, and has all his life been a working gardener; sober in his habits, conducting himself well in the affairs of life, and reported to be of pleasant manners. But, although his occupation was one which a great authority declares to be the purest of human pleasures, and the greatest refreshment to the spirits of man, it could not ward off the invasion of slowly and obscurely working causes of decay. His power of being industrious died away; his pleasant manners left him; and some months since he fell unaccountably into a state of apathy or of vague despondency; his silence only broken by moaning and lamentation; and yet retaining a capability of making a rational reply to words directly addressed to him. The good form of the head; the shape, especially, of the anterior and upper head, and the submissive expression of the features, where we find no trace of violent passions or of evil habits, are distinctly marked. We read the clear impress in the whole face of an honest man. But the eye is sunken into the socket; the grey hair hangs straight, as is usual in age; and, although he is not very far advanced in years, the withered frame and settled hopeless look, and the general expression and attitude; the drooping head, the sight unemployed on surrounding objects, the hands resting on the thighs, and the mental revelations of the eyelids, and of the forehead, and of the protruded under-lip; with the line drawn from the angle of the nose to the mouth, as well that line of age and care drawing down the corner of the mouth itself: all convey to the student of the human face, that, with failing nutrition hope has failed also; that the patient has come to a conclu-

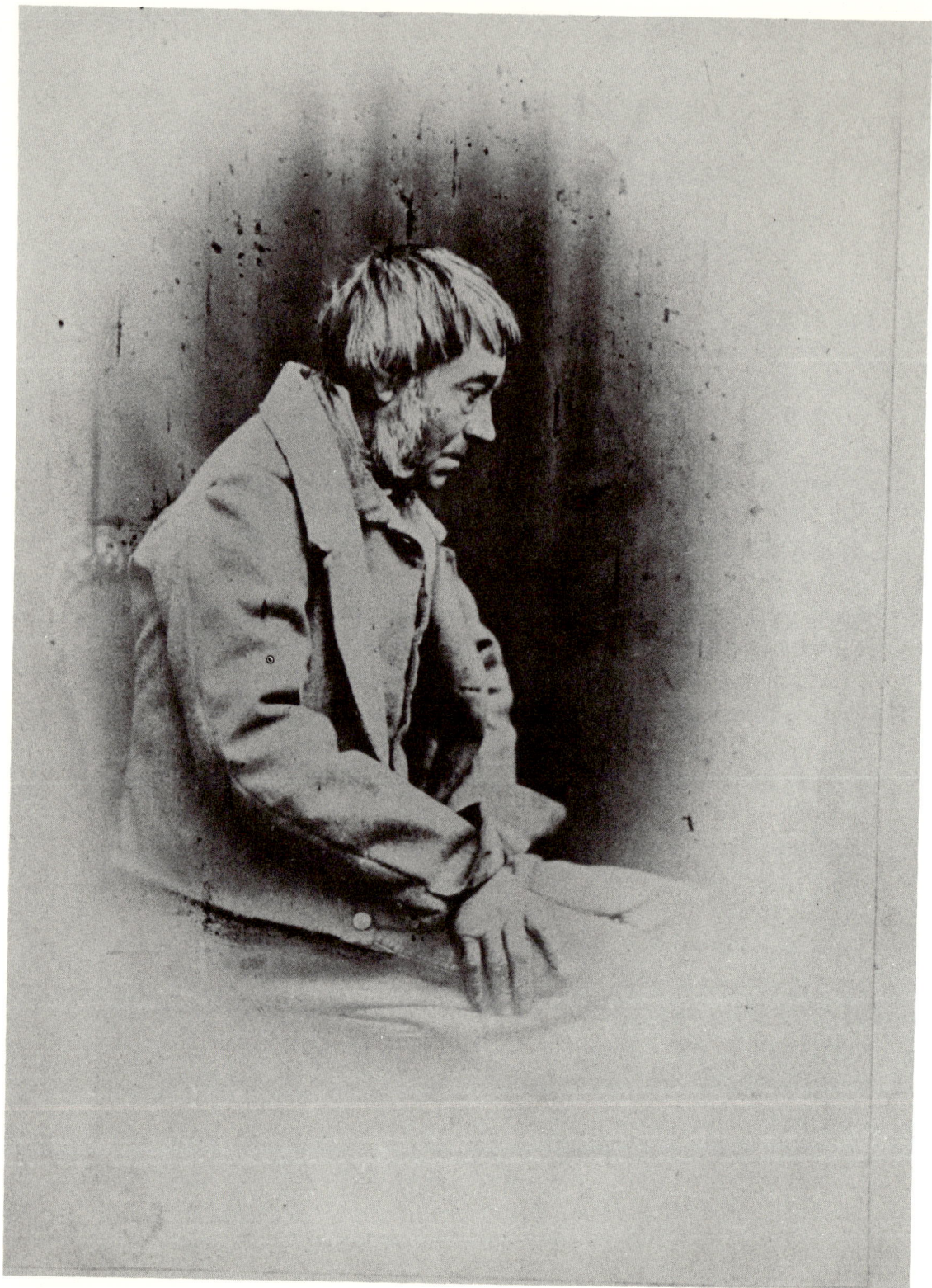

PLATE 5

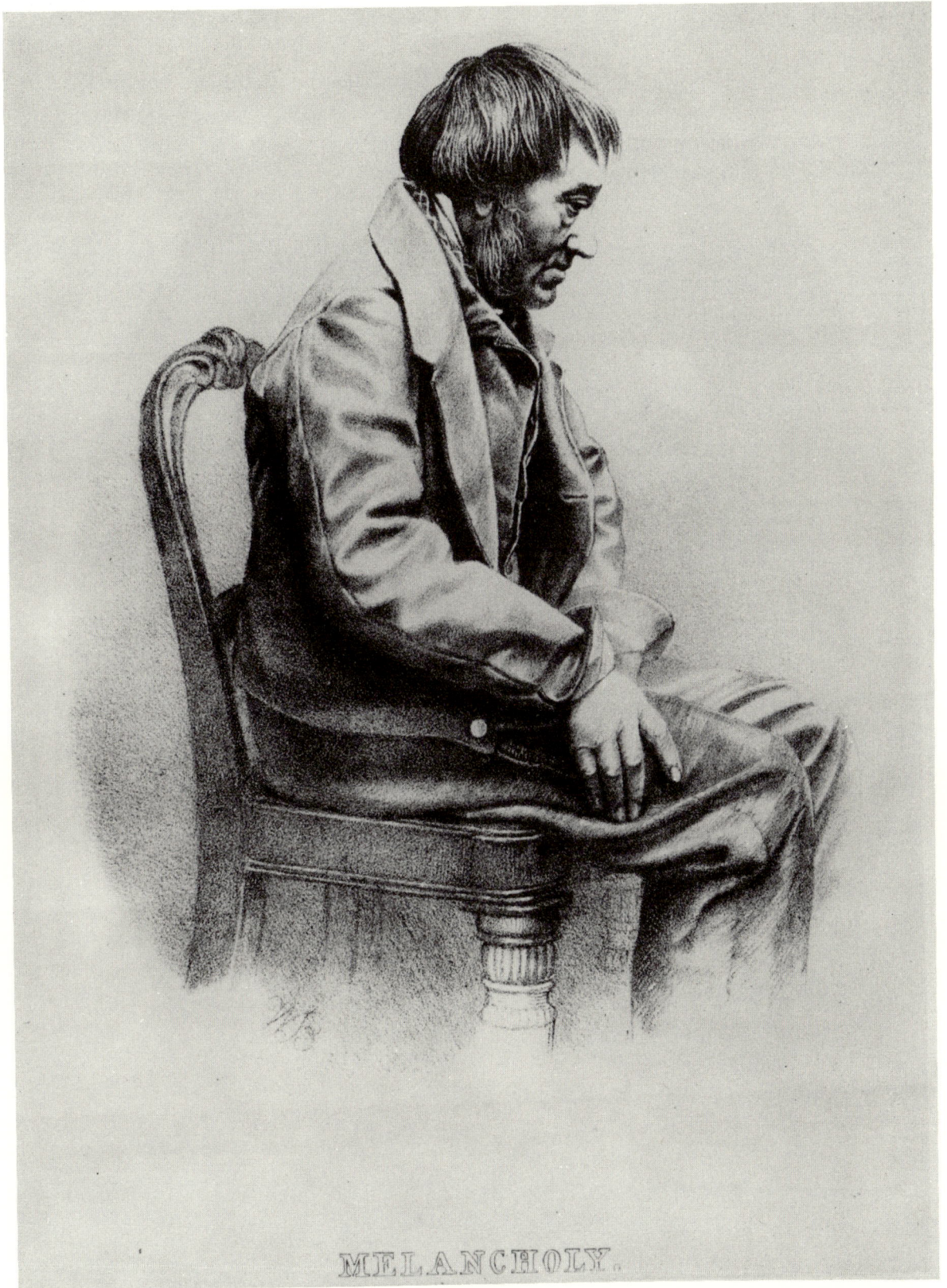

MELANCHOLY.

PLATE 6

sion that insuperable trouble has fallen upon him, and that, ever meditating upon this, still he finds no way to escape. Dulness, therefore, the advancing shadow of the dulness of death, rests upon him, never in this world to be withdrawn.

In the engraving from the photograph accompanying the present paper, there will be found certain modifications of action of the muscles of the face differing from those in the three preceding ones; as in the present instance the patient, after being insane some months, and then falling into utter despondency, and continuing in that state for a month, was in a transition state towards mania. Her story is but one in a larger chapter of such which London furnishes. She gained a small livelihood by the occupation of a sorter and folder of paper, and lived but poorly. After a confinement she had an attack of puerperal mania, lasting about six months; her conversation was generally incoherent, and her actions were sometimes impulsive and violent. She repudiated her infant, declaring that it did not belong to her, and on one occasion she leaped out of a window fourteen feet from the ground. About a month after being received into the Surrey Asylum the excitement left her, and great despondency supervened. She then sat all day in one position, or else stood up covering her face with her hands. She never employed herself, and would not reply when spoken to. For many months she remained in this state, and then what at first appeared to be recovery took place, and her faculties seemed to revive. The melancholia, however, soon returned, and continud six months more. Then, a sudden renewal of bodily and mental energy occurred, and she became maniacal; began to dress herself fantastically, sung songs, and indulged in various ideas connected with wealth and pleasure, in which state she at present remains. The photograph, taken when the state of melancholy was passing into that of excitement, retains something of the fixedness of attitude and expression in the first state; as in the arms held close to the body, and the position of the lower extremities, and in the downward tension of the cheek. The body is thin, and the hair is lank and heavy. But the eyes are not lost in vacancy; they seem to discern some person or object which excites

JOHN CONOLLY

45

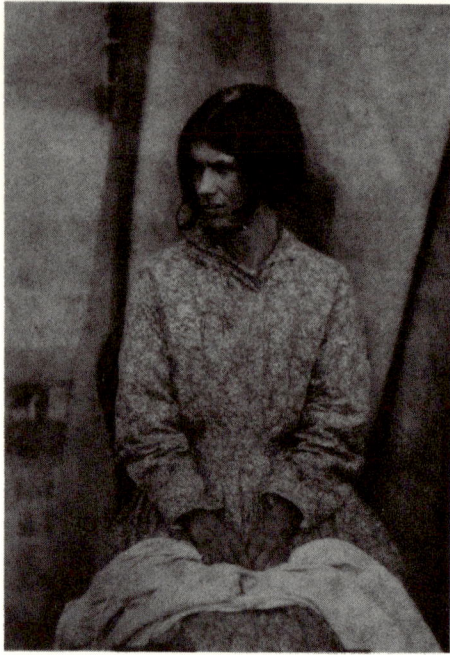

PLATE 7

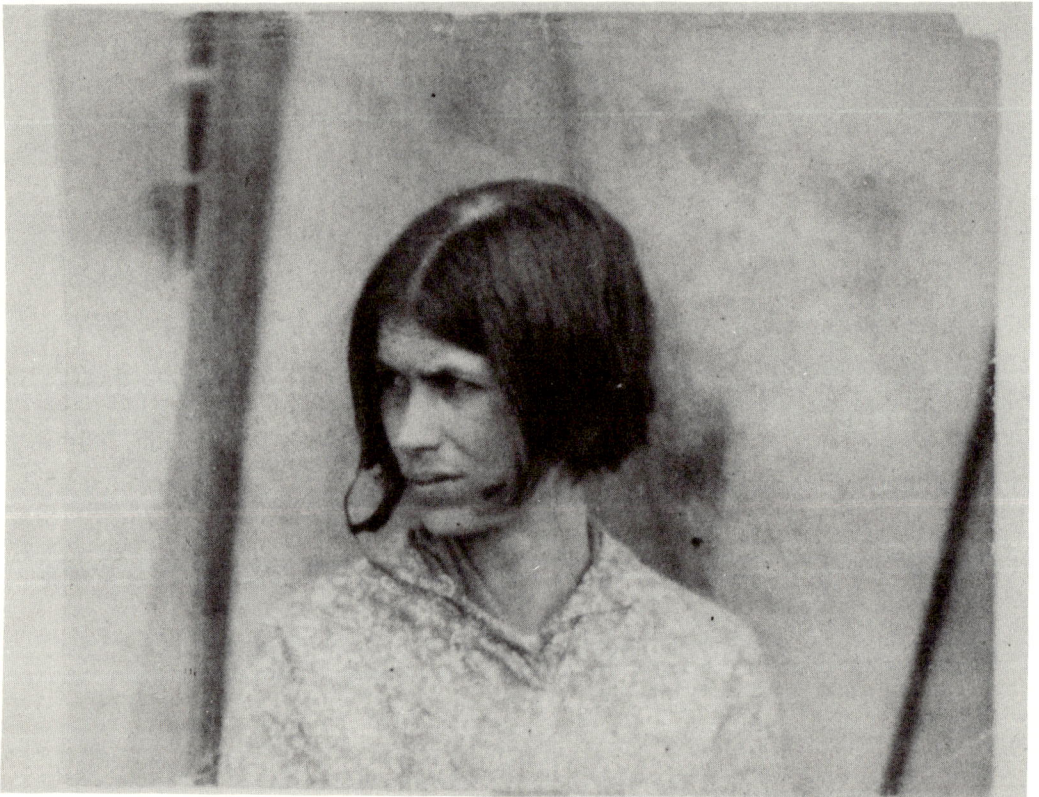

PLATE 8

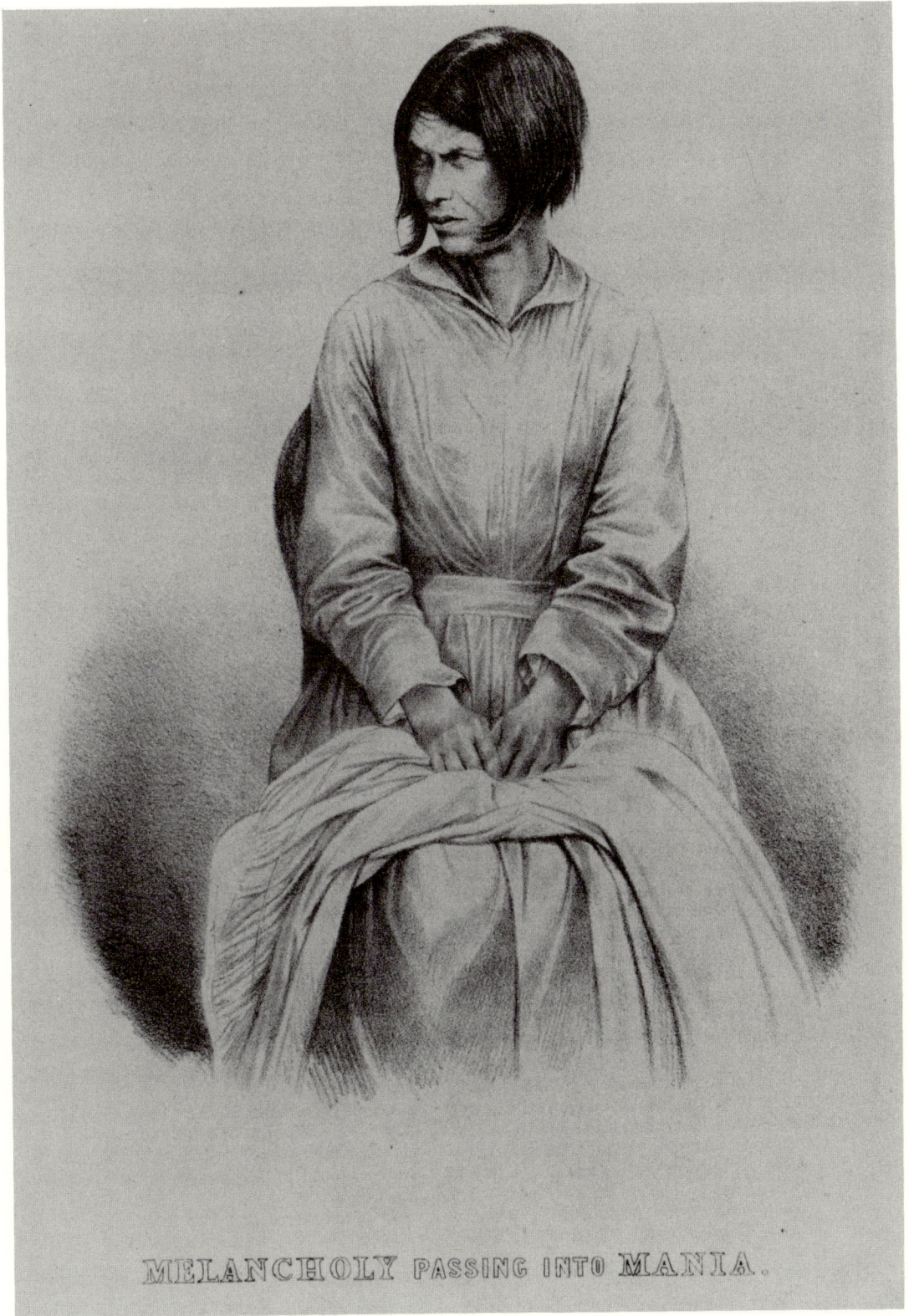

MELANCHOLY PASSING INTO MANIA.

PLATE 9

displeasure or suspicion. The forehead is wrinkled with some strong emotion, and the eyebrows, although corrugated, have not the tense contraction toward the nose which is observable in many cases of melancholia. The lips are not drawn down at the angles, but, although well shaped, are somewhat compressed, and the lower jaw indicates some half-formed determination. The maniacal condition of this patient has been accompanied with such an increase of stoutness that subsequent photographs are scarcely to be recognised as being likenesses of the same patient. Her face has become broad; the angles of the mouth are a little drawn up, giving it an expression of merriment; her forehead is smooth, the hair is well arranged, and the eyes and eyebrows are significant of animated observation, whilst the whole attitude is perfectly free from constraint.

PLATES 10 & 11

In . . . the present number, we have a specimen of the odd characters found among the older inmates of asylums, and which, before this series of papers is concluded, must have, as they deserve, a chapter to themselves. Comical as this picture of an old woman appears at the first view, it tells a somewhat lamentable tale of long mental vexation; supervening probably among the trials of the middle or even the youthful period of life, when carelessness, unheeded or untended, a giddy mind uneducated, wild manners and irregular habits, unrestrained by any care or protection, opened a wide way to disturbance: or when perhaps frequent want, or constant discomfort, and wild disorder, or the sharper sorrows incidental even to almost homeless classes of people, unsettled the intellect altogether. The apparently careless air, the reversed bonnet, and a sort of drollery lurking in the cheeks and chin, are largely mixed with traces both of former agitation and excitement, and also with some shadows of lost hope and joy. Activity, and a certain strength of character seem depicted in the general form of the face; in the well-formed forehead, wide and high; in the broad and pronounced chin; in the development of the superciliary region of the brow, and, perhaps, even in the nose. One feels sure that once this poor woman was of a merry mind, and danced and sang, and turned her bonnet round for very mirth. Even now there is something in the position of her head and her general attitude which betokens a consciousness of being an odd and amusing object presented to the casual visitor; but the delvings of care in the forehead and in the whole face are still many and deep: the strong descending lines from the alae nasi to the depressed corners of the mouth, speak of alternations of depression with excitement, and make the physiognomy indicative of past attacks of mania and melancholia, both of which have left their traces there.

This odd facial expression, and the combination of various expressions, seem, indeed, to be the natural results of what was known to

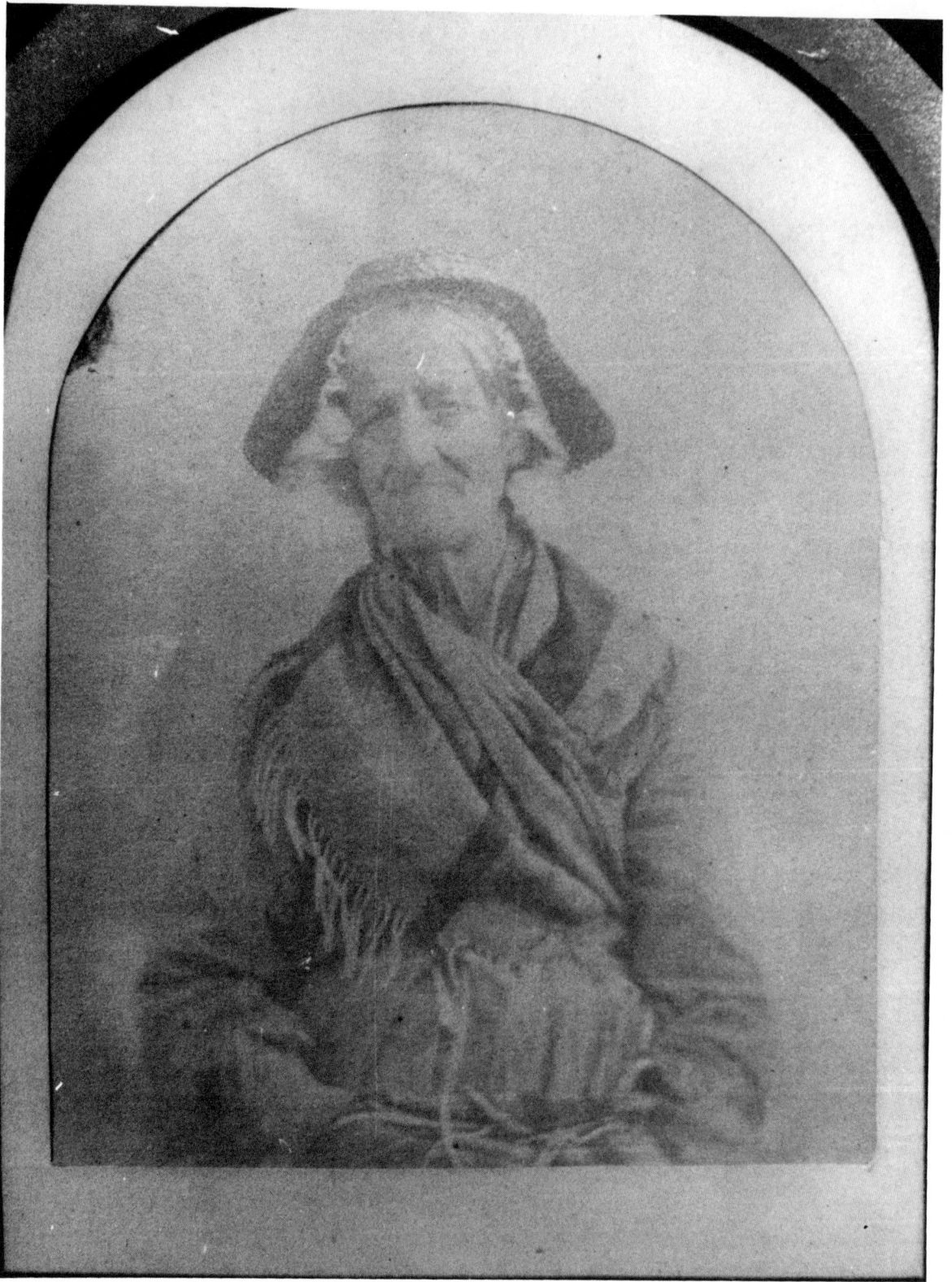

PLATE 10

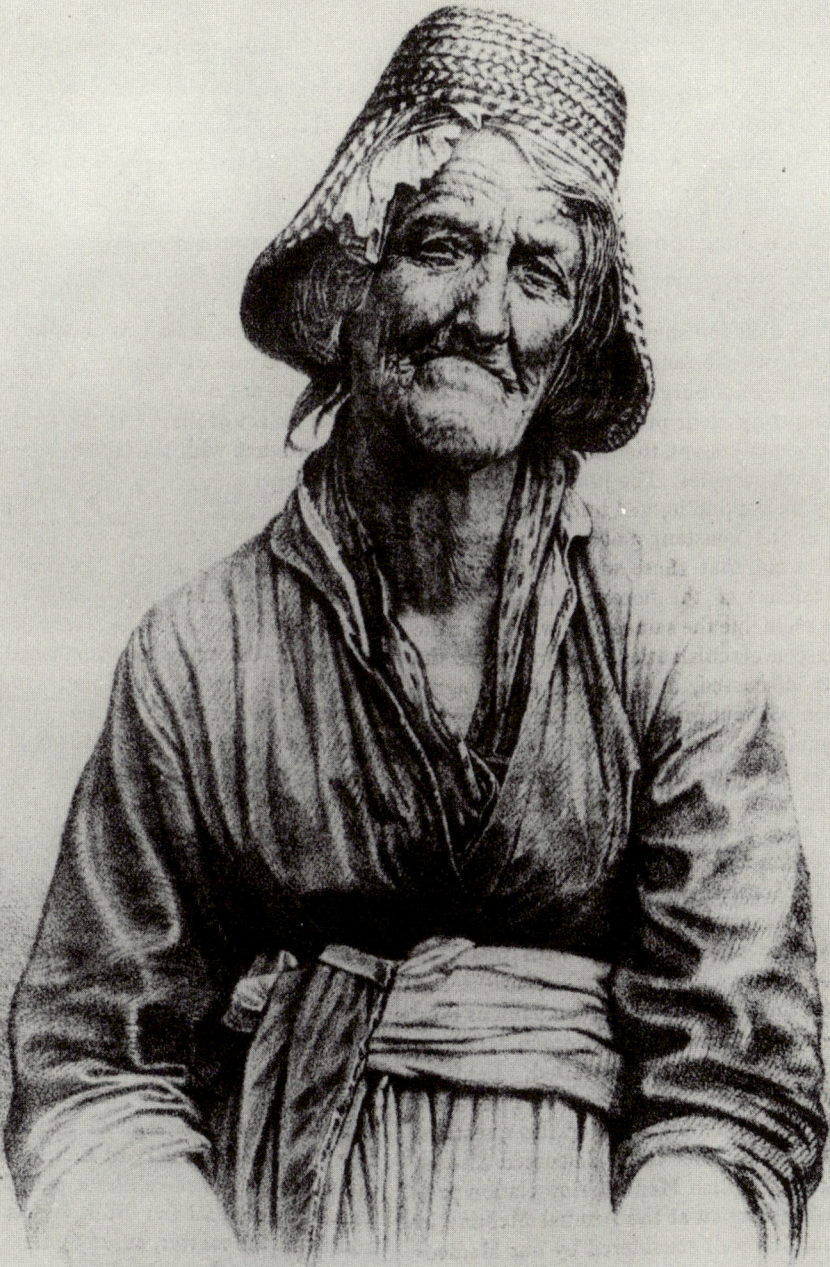

CHRONIC MANIA.

PLATE 11

have been her mode of life. She was by occupation a washerwoman, and, no doubt, for a time active and hard-working. Advancing to middle age, and beginning to feel the exhaustion incidental to daily labour, she began to seek the resource of temporary stimulants, and, soothed and stupefied with gin, became less and less careful as to food, or to food of a good description: for gin seems to silence hunger as it silences conscience. She became occasionally violent, and at length unmanageable except in an asylum; to which she was taken seventeen years ago. The regular life led there, the good food, the general regulations of the place, and occasional Medical treatment, had their usual good effects. In the laundries of our large asylums near London such cases abound. You see a number of active women, busy at the washing-tub, or dexterous in mangling and folding, but whose air and manner, and somewhat fiery countenance, show that they are not always so composed; and, indeed, the nerves of visitors are generally more likely to be shaken in the crowd of these useful but eccentric laundresses than elsewhere; for it is the custom of many of them, on some sudden impulse, to break off from work at once, and exhibit much violence of voice and gesture. Formerly the nurses, as excited as the patients, used to overpower them and carry them off by main force to the refractory ward, in their progress to which their shouts and remonstrances diffused alarm over nearly the whole building. They are now understood much better. The peculiar form and duration of such outbreaks in these hard-working women are quite familiar to the head-laundress and her assistants; and by observing a rule of very wide application and utility in managing asylums, — the rule of letting them alone, — the most obstreperous among them, after satisfying her mind by the unrestrained expression of her uncontrollable anger, will resume all the activity of the washerwoman, and perhaps give no more trouble for weeks to come.

Such appears to have been the character of the old lady in the reversed bonnet. But the maniacal attack being the first she had experienced, and occurring when at a curable age — a little more than forty — the asylum-influences had a happy effect upon her, and in about eleven months she was discharged cured. But there are patients who seem, however apparently well, still to require this external influence to keep their minds rational; and this poor woman appears to have been one of them; for although it was said that she did not relapse into intemperate habits as to drinking, she was not found to be an endurable neighbour when at large, and was very soon taken back to the asylum. She has acquired the habit of taking large quantities of snuff, a fondness for which appeared to have superseded the fondness for gin; and to obtain snuff she was capable of any cunning, or sometimes of any violence. Even the habit of snuff-taking, the most difficult, it is said, of all small indulgences to be wholly abandoned, she was persuaded to give up, and with very great advantage as regarded mental tranquillity and general behaviour. Now and then fits of violence still occur; but her usual state is that of an odd, cunning, mischievous patient, delighting in eccentricity of dress.

In this Illustration we fancy that we see represented an individual on whom the oblivion of years has crept gently: one who has gone on day after day, for a great part of his life, with occupations demanding talent and accuracy, but of which he was perfectly master. By slow degrees he grew incapable of continuous attention to minutiae, now and then became puzzled, now and then forgetful, and dreamy and drowsy; wondering, meanwhile, what soporific influence was overshadowing him, and comparing himself to a man in a kind of mesmerised sleep. The figure represents a venerable ruin. In the finely-developed head we seem to read an equally well-balanced mind; without extravagance, without extremes. The eye is large and meditative, the nose well pronounced, the lower jaw indicative of steadiness and strength. In the upper lip there is, perhaps, a want of compression, belonging to the approaching dementia. The whole figure, and also the drooping eyelid, bespeak repose. It is happy for old men when this repose is seldom disturbed. Few of them are so privileged as not to feel from time to time a sort of pang of mental dissolution, or something like sensible accessions of old age, and an unavailing sorrow that all they valued perishes in this world, even as the less regarded elements of their bodies. And to mortal man such mortal experiences are real afflictions. To find the sight less acute, and the ear blunted and treacherous, and the limbs heavy, and the voice tremulous; and, worse than all, the glorious faculties of the mind gathering some strange dimness, the reflection faulty, and the imagination fickle and flighty, is to be sensible of the approaches of death; and actually to feel how gradually and yet how surely "this sensible warm motion" is becoming "a kneaded clod."

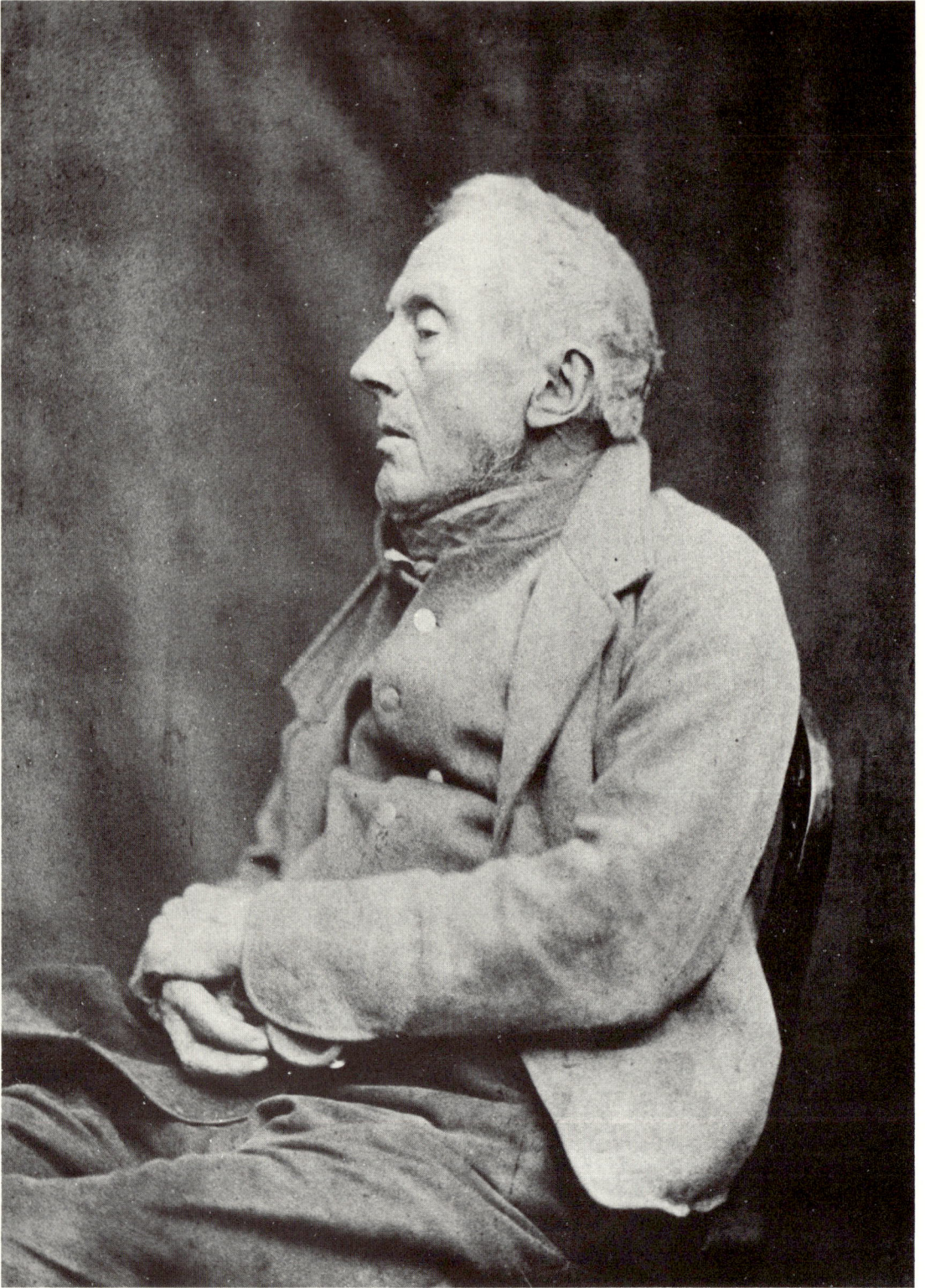

PLATE 12

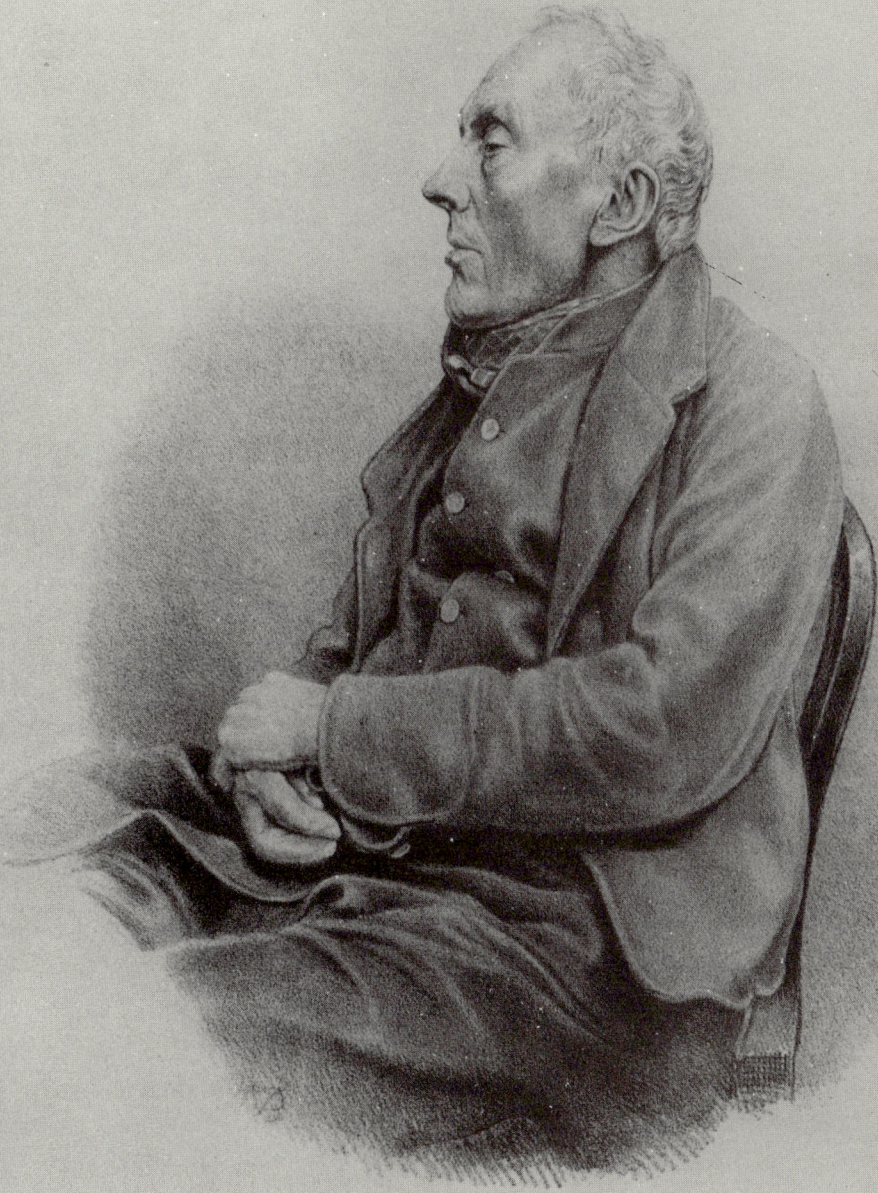

Plate 6

SENILE DEMENTIA.

From a Photograph by Dr Diamond.

PLATE 13

PLATE 14

The illustrations furnished by the admirable photographs of Dr. Diamond, and skilfully copied by the engraver, to accompany this discursive paper, present various forms of expression of face, incidental to puerperal insanity. The case thus beautifully portrayed was one of those which occasion much surprise, and even alarm, in an affectionate household. A young married woman has lately become a mother; and for some days all goes on well. The father is conscious of increased importance; the nurse is proud of the baby, and seems to consider it almost her own. But this pleasant domestic state is all at once interrupted by the altered tone, or manner, or temper of the young mother; who speaks sharply to those about her, or loses her cheerfulness, becomes indifferent to her child, and seems as if her thoughts were occupied with scenes of gaiety, or in listening to amusing conversations; adopting a levity of manner and a fantastic arrangement of her head-dress or general apparel; and seeming to be detached from her husband, and from all about her, and from everything real. This is terrible in every rank of life: among the poor it is ruinous.

In the *first* of the four portraits of a case of this kind, there is represented a short initial stage of dulness and apathy. The patient was very quiet, and even sullen when addressed: she remained nearly all day in one posture, her hands crossed and resting on her knees, after the manner of melancholic patients; but the countenance, it will be seen, rather expresses bewilderment than unmixed depression; the eyes are directed forward; there is no very marked drawing down of the corner of the mouth or of the chin, and there is a slight elevation of the upper part of the cheeks; altogether, rather indicative of some advancing reverie, more agreeable than talk, or even than food; and this patient was indeed not only sullen when spoken to, but refused food, partly, perhaps, because she feared to abandon the reverie.

There was, however, a depression mingled with her reveries, arising, as it would appear, from real circumstances. She had been an industrious woman, of good character; but she and her husband were poor, and, contemplating, probably, the difficulty of providing food, and clothes, and shelter for a coming family, her husband left her, and his home, and his country, to seek employment in Australia. The sensitive wife, whose mother had been insane, became deranged and melancholic, almost as soon as her poor little child came into the world of want, in which the father was so perplexed how to provide against starvation. But in a few days the memory of real events died away, and the malady assumed the form most generally seen after delivery. All the harassing troubles of life were forgotten, and husband and baby and her lonely home. The *second* portrait was taken eight days after the first. Her features were then not only lively, but mirthful; the mouth is drawn out laterally, the nostrils are expanded, and the lively eyes, the elevated eyebrows, and the merry cheeks and chin are felicitously rendered in the plate. She still sits with her hands crossed, and resting on her knee; but she looks as if she might easily be persuaded to get up and dance. She was, indeed generally singing; she tore her clothes out of an excess of animal spirits; and she now took food, not only willingly but voraciously.

In about six weeks from the commencement of the malady, a great change took place, and recovery seemed to commence. She became quite comfortable, and was employed in needlework; but had a somewhat impatient desire to go away from the asylum. At this time the *third* portrait was taken. She is seen standing up, and neatly dressed. Her face has lost its broad merriment; but there is a tension of the facial muscles, which prevents the experienced Physician from concluding that all the malady has yet passed away. Perfect muscular composure has not yet been established. In accordance with these prognostics, in a fortnight afterward she relapsed into the state of drollery and destructiveness portrayed in the second portrait. Happily, the relapse was only temporary, and in ten days more she was again industrious, and quite tranquil. From this time she remained so; and when her recovery was confirmed by a month or two more of observation, which the relapse had made advisable, she left the asylum quite well, — an event commemorated by the *fourth* portrait, wherein

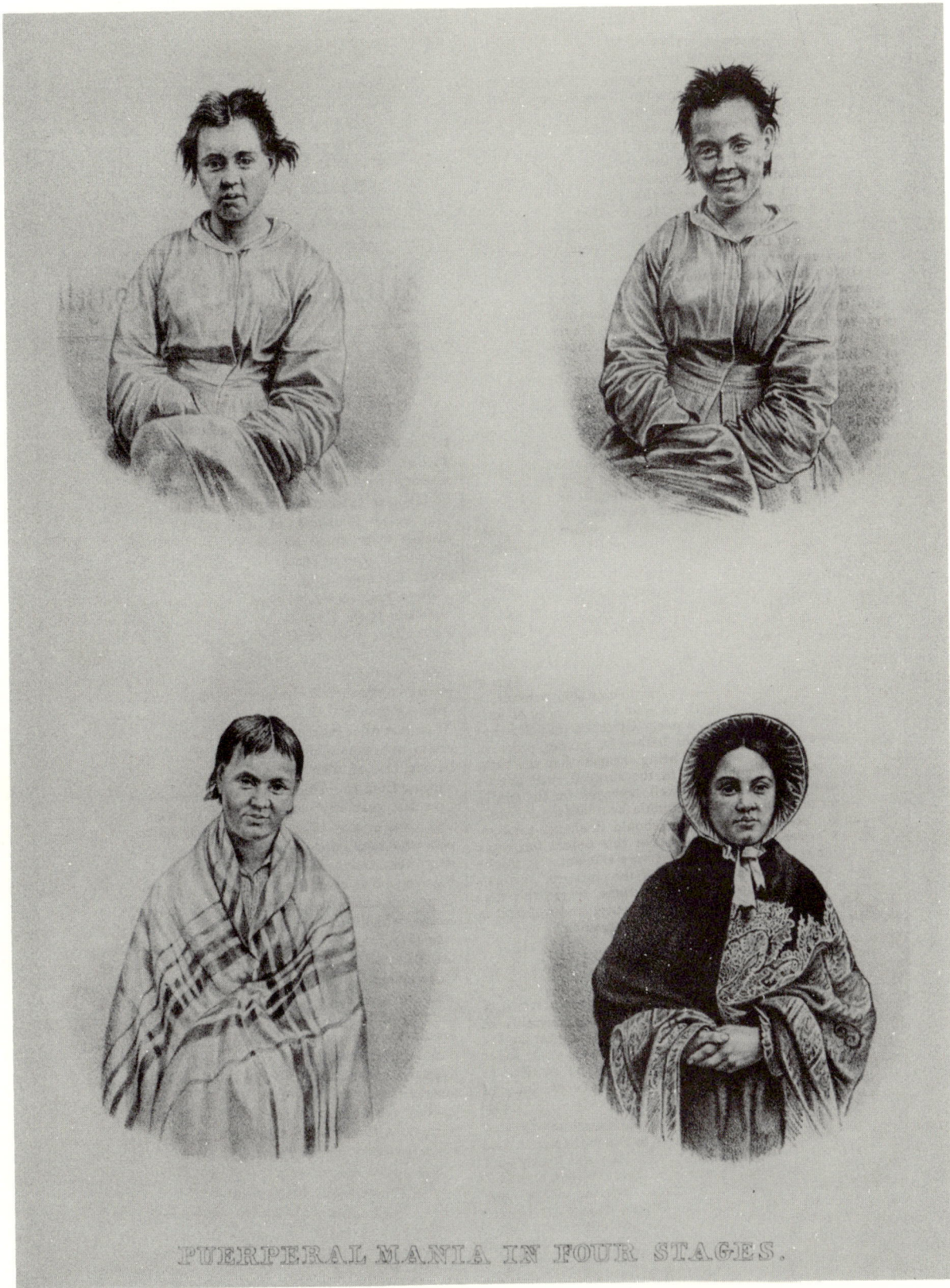

PUERPERAL MANIA IN FOUR STAGES.

PLATE 14

she is represented in bonnet and shawl, with composed features and pleasant honest face, animated still, but no longer excited; her general appearance indicating the restoration of the health and strength to be sufficiently called upon in the undertaking now meditated, of taking out her baby and rejoining her poor husband in Australia.

PLATE 15

At first this was a case of puerperal mania, with a propensity to suicide. Melancholia succeeded to this stage, and after a time gave place to a return of maniacal excitement. The portrait represents the patient in the transition stage from sadness to renewed excitement. Although the melancholy traces of the form of her malady in its first stage have not wholly disappeared, new emotions have evidently risen up in the mind, and have modified the movements of the muscles of the face. The lines of care from the alae of the nose remain, and the chin and lower part of the cheek still retain the impress of depression; but the eyes have awakened from the gloomy sleep of the melancholic stage, and are bent energetically, even fiercely, on some real or imaginary object, near or distant. The forehead, still wrinkled, bespeaks aroused attention; and the general expression of the face is that of an angry sense of injury inflicted, and of some novel suspicions which menace violent actions. The patient, it will be remembered, was subjected to the photographer when mania was displacing the melancholia to which it had previously given way. There are many patients whose mental disorder, being incurable, presents these alternations several times in a year, and for all the remaining years of life. An unhappy man will pace up and down some chosen part of the ward of an Asylum, or of the gravel-walk of a garden, day after day, for many months, until the very earth and stones are worn; never speaking, never smiling; the personification of misery. But to this state may succeed a strangely-contrasted gaiety, lively talking, wild laughter, and the dance of merriment. Unhappy-looking women, who have sat from morning to night, week after week, the hands clasped and pressed on the breast; the eyes heedless of the passers by; and dependent on the help of attendants as respected dress, food, and every other care; pass from this moping condition to a state of gaiety which produces amusement even among their fellow-patients; unex-

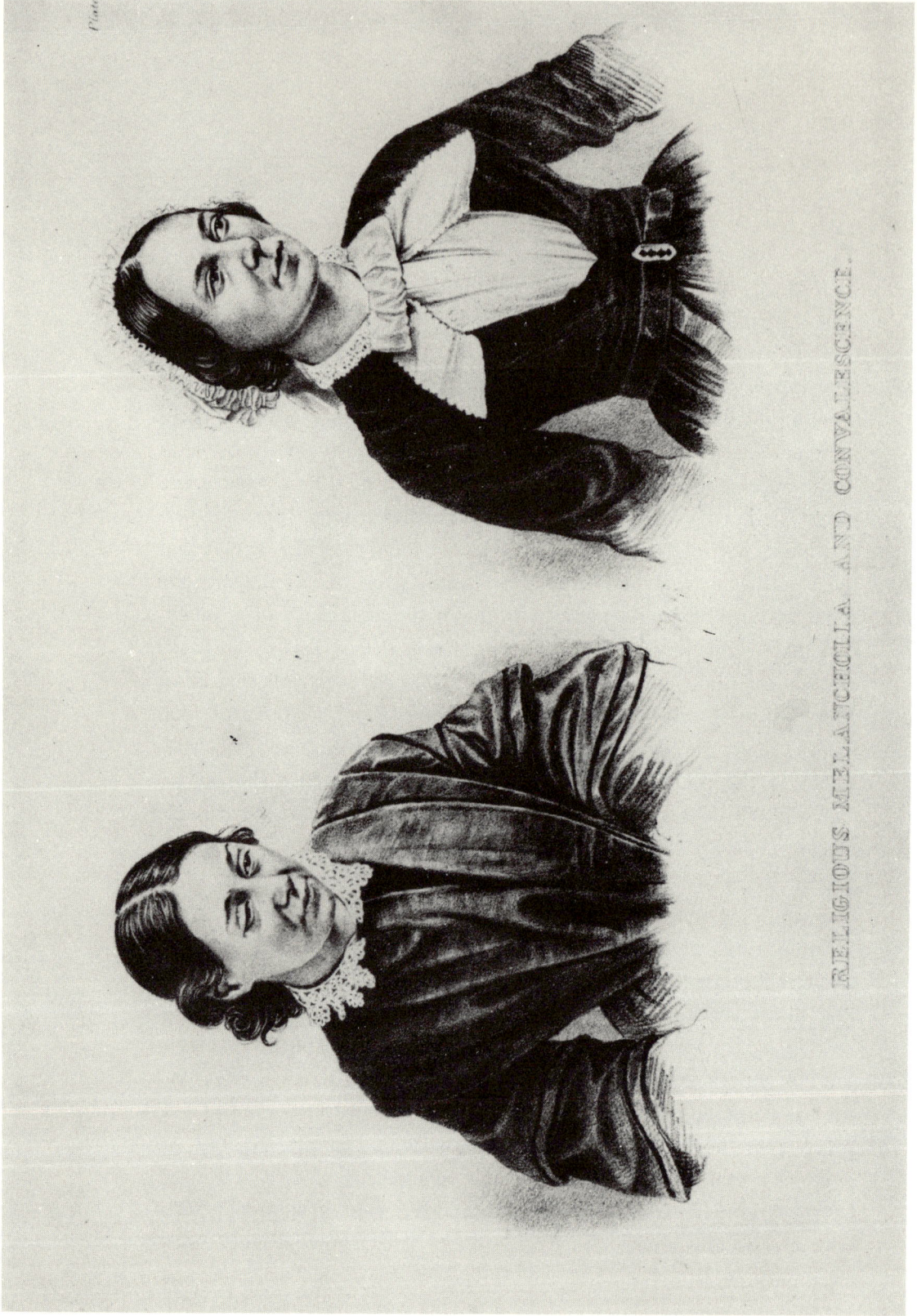

RELIGIOUS MELANCHOLIA AND CONVALESCENCE.

PLATE 15

pectedly making their appearance in some old and carefully preserved finery; their hair curled and ornamented; their whole deportment displaying the vanity of fancied beauty and of faded grace marvellously restored.

PLATES 16 & 17

The portraits accompanying this paper are illustrative of some of the modifications of features and expression in women who have fallen into habits of intemperance, on which derangement of the mental powers has ensued to a greater or less extent. The two portraits represent different patients, of different character and of different history. The poor creature on the right [Plate 17] having been nurtured in low life, almost brought up in early acquired habits of drinking, left to do their sure and uninterrupted work on body and mind until both have acquired the impress of a misfortune unavoidable, and slowly ripened into vice, and bringing the whole creature into a sort of chronic and indelible appearance of sottishness. In the left-hand portrait is represented another patient, of a respectable station in life, but also ruined by drink; but by drink so gradually indulged in, however, that her altered state bewilders her, and fills her, fallen as she is, with distressful remorse.

Although we perceive even in this portrait the somewhat bloated or swollen condition of the fleshy parts of the face which tipsy habits produce, much expression remains — but it is of wretchedness and despair. The raised hands, pressed together, indicate the intensity of her prominent emotions; the eyes somewhat uplifted, but gazing on nothing; the deep corrugation of the overhanging integuments of the lower forehead, portray the painful questioning of a woman not forgetful of her former life, nor unconscious of the comfortless change that has come over her; and the expression is heightened by those undefinable modifications of the muscular structure of the cheeks which add so much to all facial expression of intense character. In the upraised under lip, also, and in the tensely-elevated chin, there is so much meaning of the same kind, that we might almost fancy the poor patient breaking out, in this suffering mood, into expressive words, as was indeed the poor woman's custom often, relative to her earlier life now gone, and happier thoughts long dispersed, and to remembrances

JOHN CONOLLY

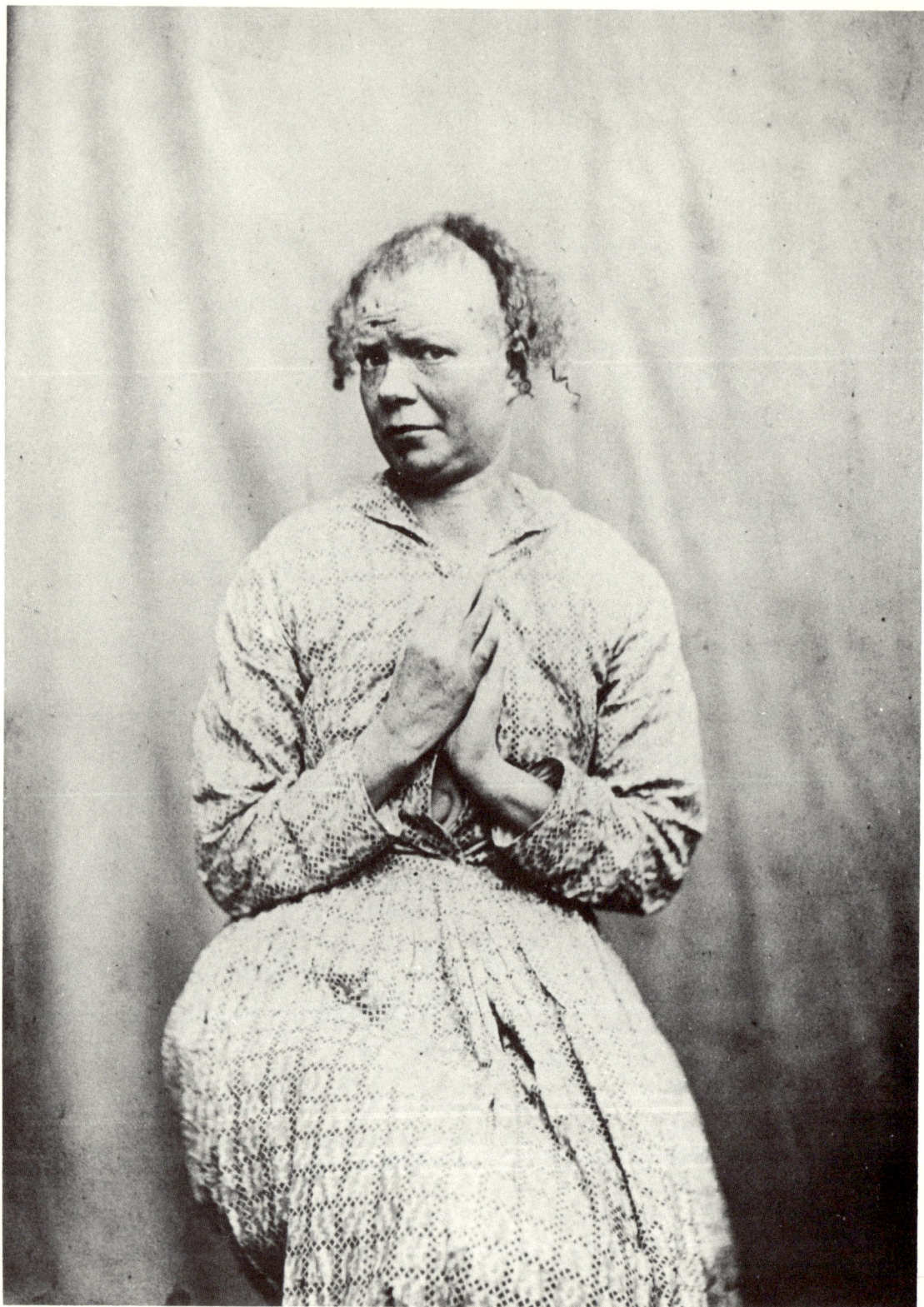

PLATE 16

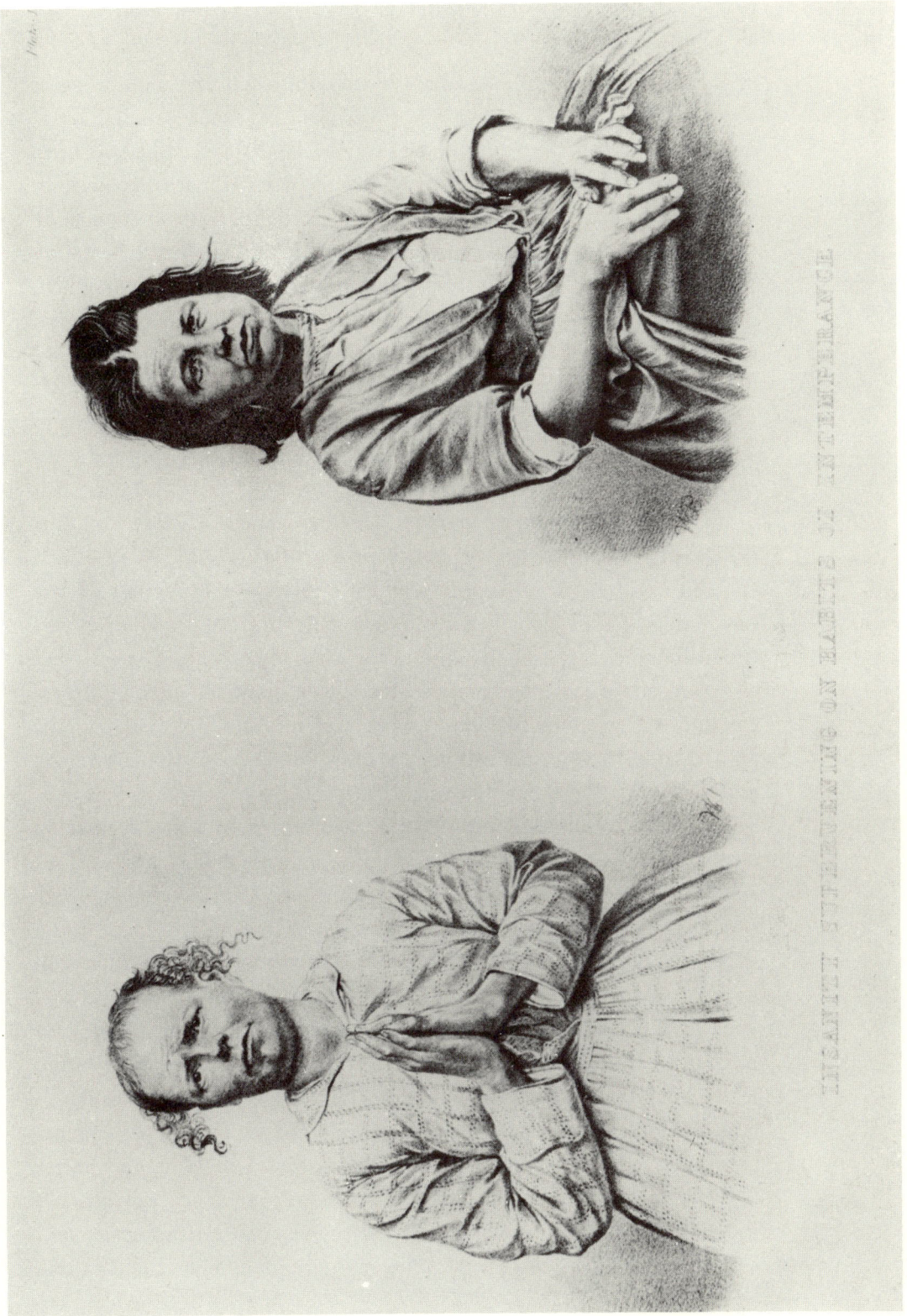

INSANITY SUPERVENING IN STATES OF EXTEMPERANCE

PLATE 17

of having once been esteemed and even admired in the modest circle in which she moved, until taught to like gin by "wicked neighbours" older than herself. Her history was indeed lamentable. She had been well educated, and resided, when a young woman, with her mother, who possessed a little independent property. Being then good looking, she was much noticed; nor did it appear that she lost her station by any immorality of early life. But she was not watched enough to guard her from pernicious acquaintances, who enjoyed, it would seem, the perverse satisfaction of teaching her the poor pleasures arising from the taste of spirituous liquors, until she adopted Mrs. Gamp's plan of putting gin into the teapot. Somehow, as always happens in such cases, the little property possessed by her mother gradually diminished, and at length disappeared altogether. Dram-drinking became the only remaining comfort of the impoverished house; and thus things went on until one article of furniture after another, and also the clothes of her mother and herself, passed into the hands of the pawnbrokers. The poor mother found shelter in the workhouse, and the still more unhappy daughter, torn by remorse, and maddened more and more by intemperance now grown habitual, became maniacal, and was received into the lunatic asylum. Much of this, perhaps all of it, is written in that despairing, questioning face. Memory of the past and purer time has not been destroyed by her malady, nor conscience obliterated. She feels herself transformed, and that for her no earthly joy remains or will return. Her irritable hands have traced marks of agony on her forehead; her neglected curls hang raggedly over her ears; she has torn them away until she is nearly bald. Even her large and well-developed brain seems to impress the beholder with thoughts aggravative of the miserable desolation that now alone prevails in the depths of her consciousness and memory. There is no healthful action and no comfort in any corner of that restless brain. Where once there was quick perception, imagination, benevolence, understanding, there is now but a tumultuous succession of ineffaceable records, read by the light of madness only, with no ray of better light from the retrospection, and as yet no higher hope. Suicide, the last resource of such wretchedness, has been often attempted by her. When all this affliction falls upon an erring human being, the comforts and even the blessings accorded to our poorer lunatics show all the value of the noble institutions where the most rejected of the world meet with pity and find rest. The malady may be too deeply fixed to be curable; but all physical excess is at an end — no neglect and no cruelty add to the morbid wretchedness; kind words are heard, and religious thoughts are gradually introduced into the mind of the sufferers; and the curtain of death falls gently even upon them.

A different history from the preceding is plainly enough written in the second portrait, which exhibits traits scarcely quite unknown to persons accustomed to the observation of the faces of populous towns. Here the bloated face, the pendulous masses of cheek, the large lips uncontrolled by any voluntary expression, and to which refinement and delicacy seem never to have belonged; the heavily gazing eyes, not speculative, scarcely conscious; the disordered, uncombed, capriciously cut hair, cut with ancient scissors or chopped with impatient knife; the indolent position of the body, and the heavy resting of the coarse, unemployed, outstretched fingers, together with the neglected dress and reckless *abandon* of the patient, all concur to declare the woman of low and degraded life, into whose mind, even before madness supervened, no thoughts except gross thoughts were wont to enter; and whose bold eye and prominent mouth were never, even from early infancy, employed to express any of the higher or softer sensibilities of a woman's soul. But yet she is, even in this degraded state, more truly an object of pity than of condemnation. It is easy to condemn; — it is harder to be just. Where this now outcast human being was born, and how brought up, it were vain to inquire. She probably never had a home; and it appears, in fact, that her earliest reminiscences were only of gaining a kind of livelihood by selling miscellaneous articles in the streets; articles begged, or articles lent, or articles stolen, no doubt. As she grew up, gross appetites grew up also; the love of beer, among the rest, developed itself strongly; and she was well known to her familiars as what even they denominated a low-lived person. But beer was sometimes hard to procure; it could not always be successfuly begged for; it could not be easily stolen; and it could not be bought without money. So the want of this stimulant joy of low life caused her to cultivate her faculties as a singer, and these were exerted in low public-houses, where the remuneration was generally beer, or halfpence convertible into beer. Her audiences were not fastidious; her songs were not always unobjectionable; and she further became liable to infirmities of temper, and acquired habits of inconvenient violence; became signalised for artful frauds and cunning concealments, and in all respects negligent in her habits. At last she was pronounced to be insane, and found refuge, the only refuge in this world, from worldly misery, in an asylum; but she could scarcely appreciate even the comforts of an asylum. The beds and the clothing might be good, and the food; but the limitation of beer constituted a permanent grievance.

PLATES 18–54

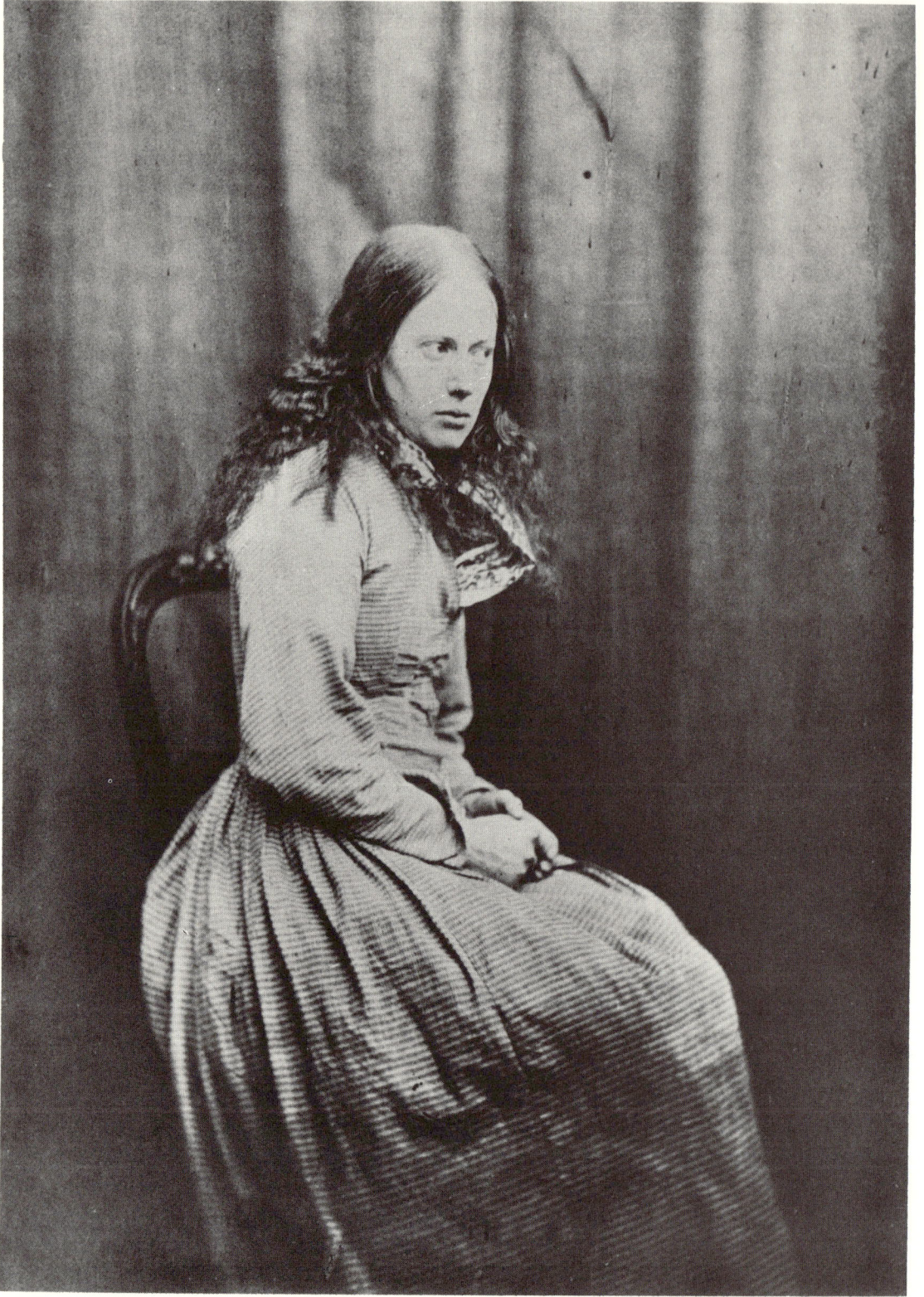

PLATE 18

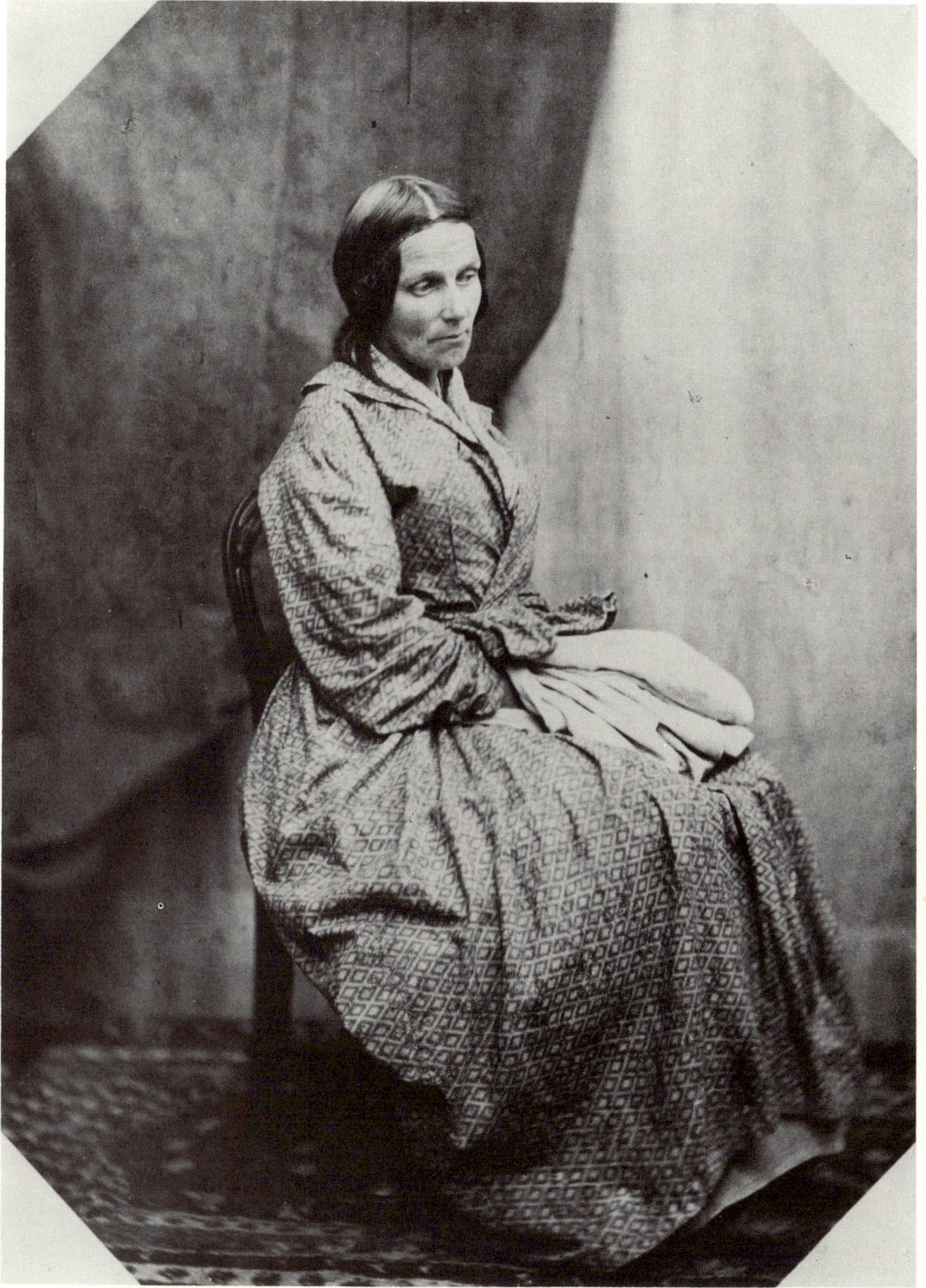

PLATE 19

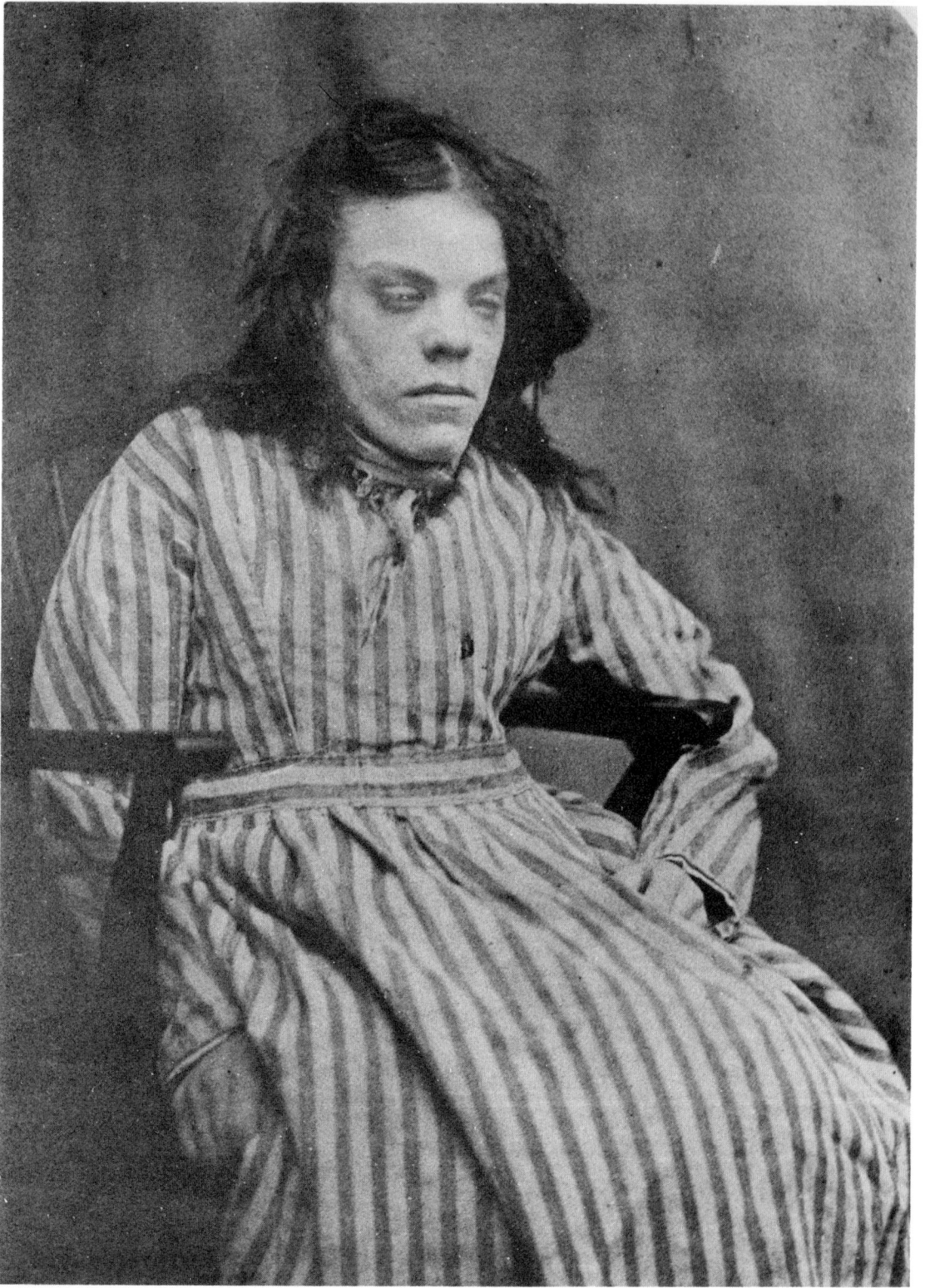

PLATE 20

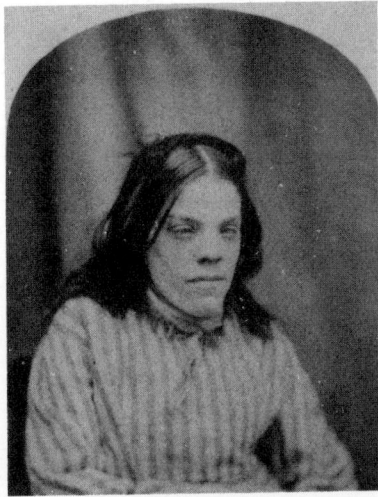

PLATE 21

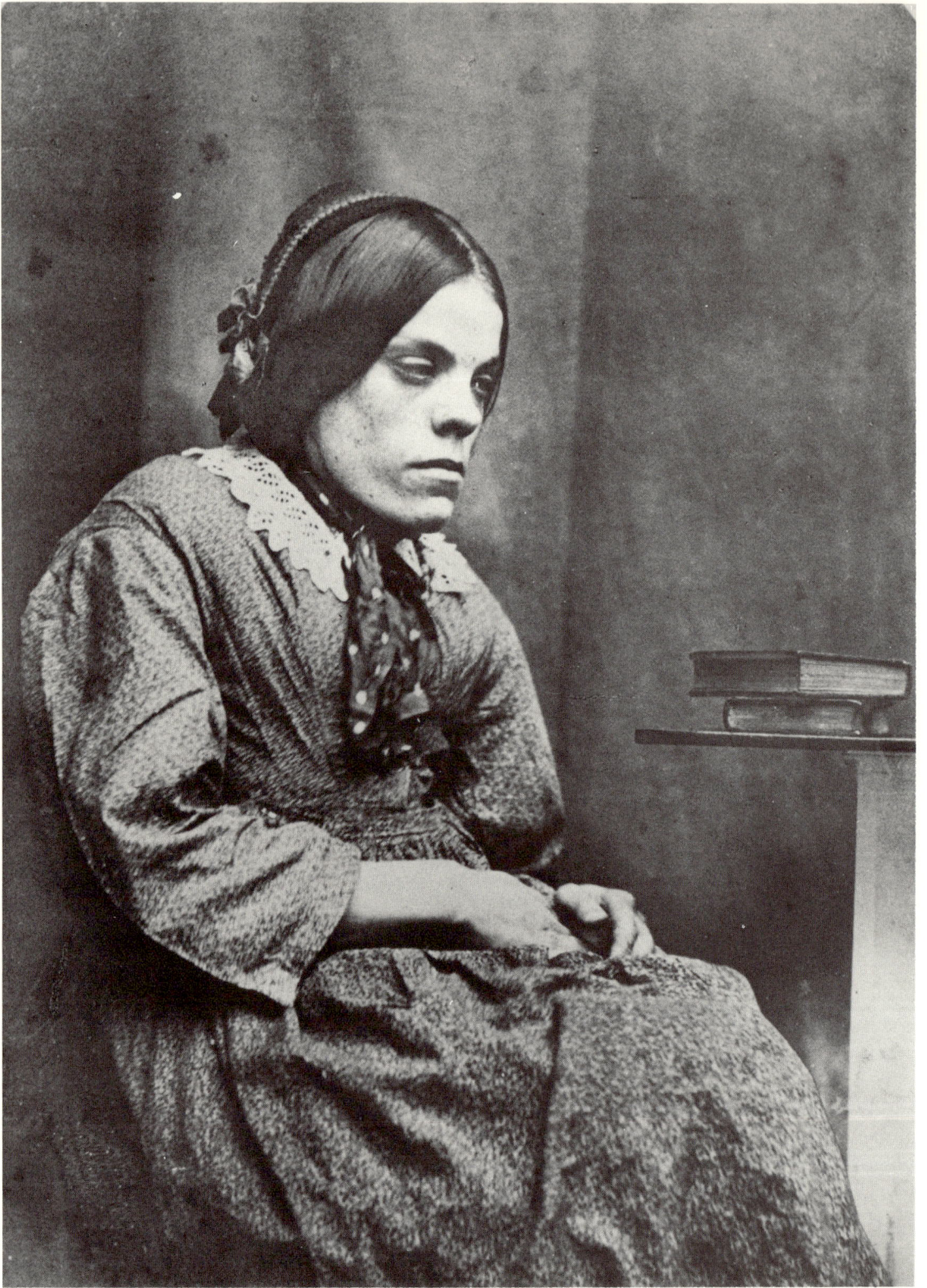

PLATE 22

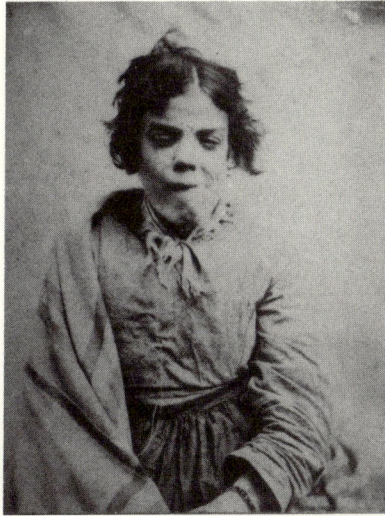

PLATE 23

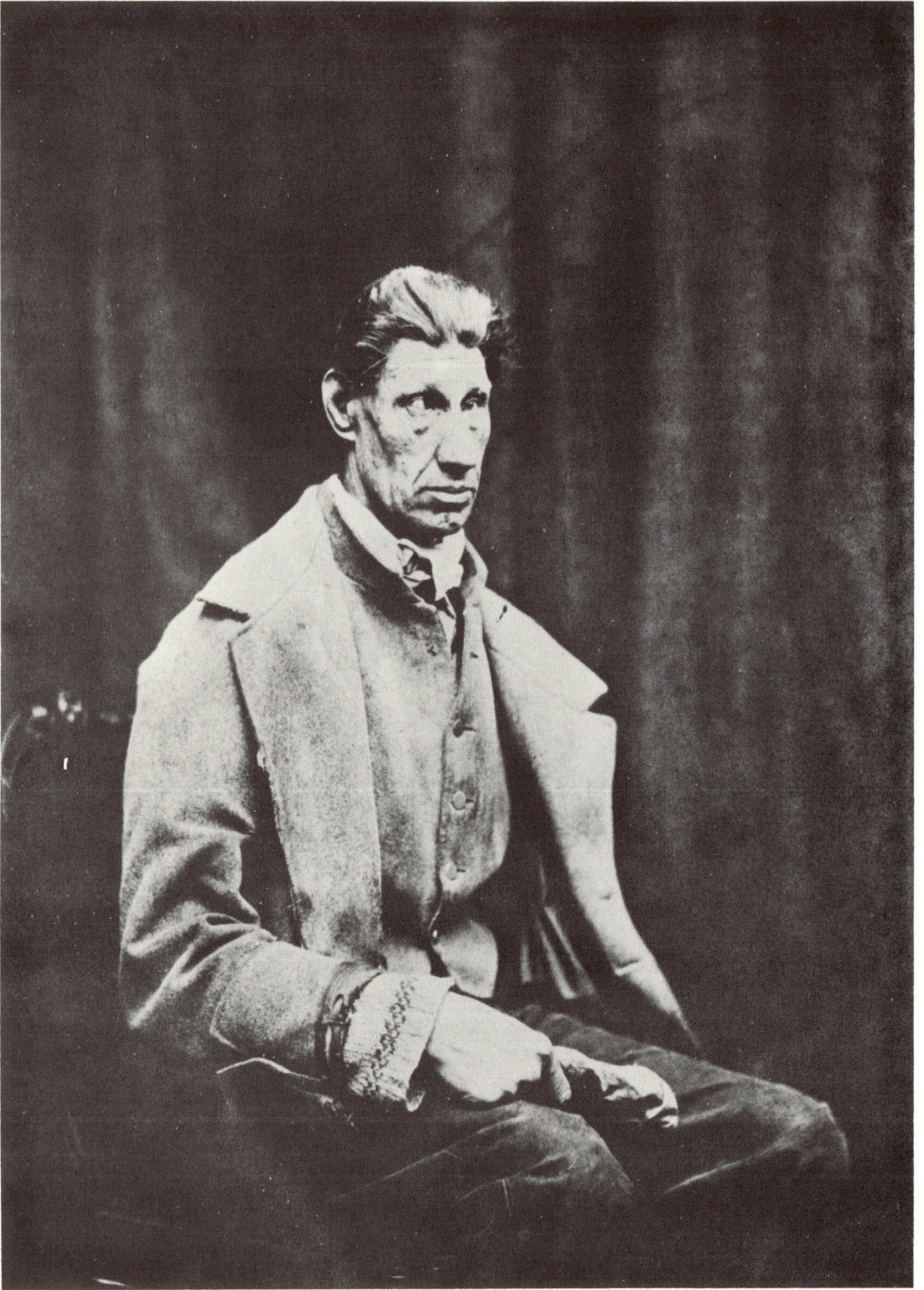

PLATE 24

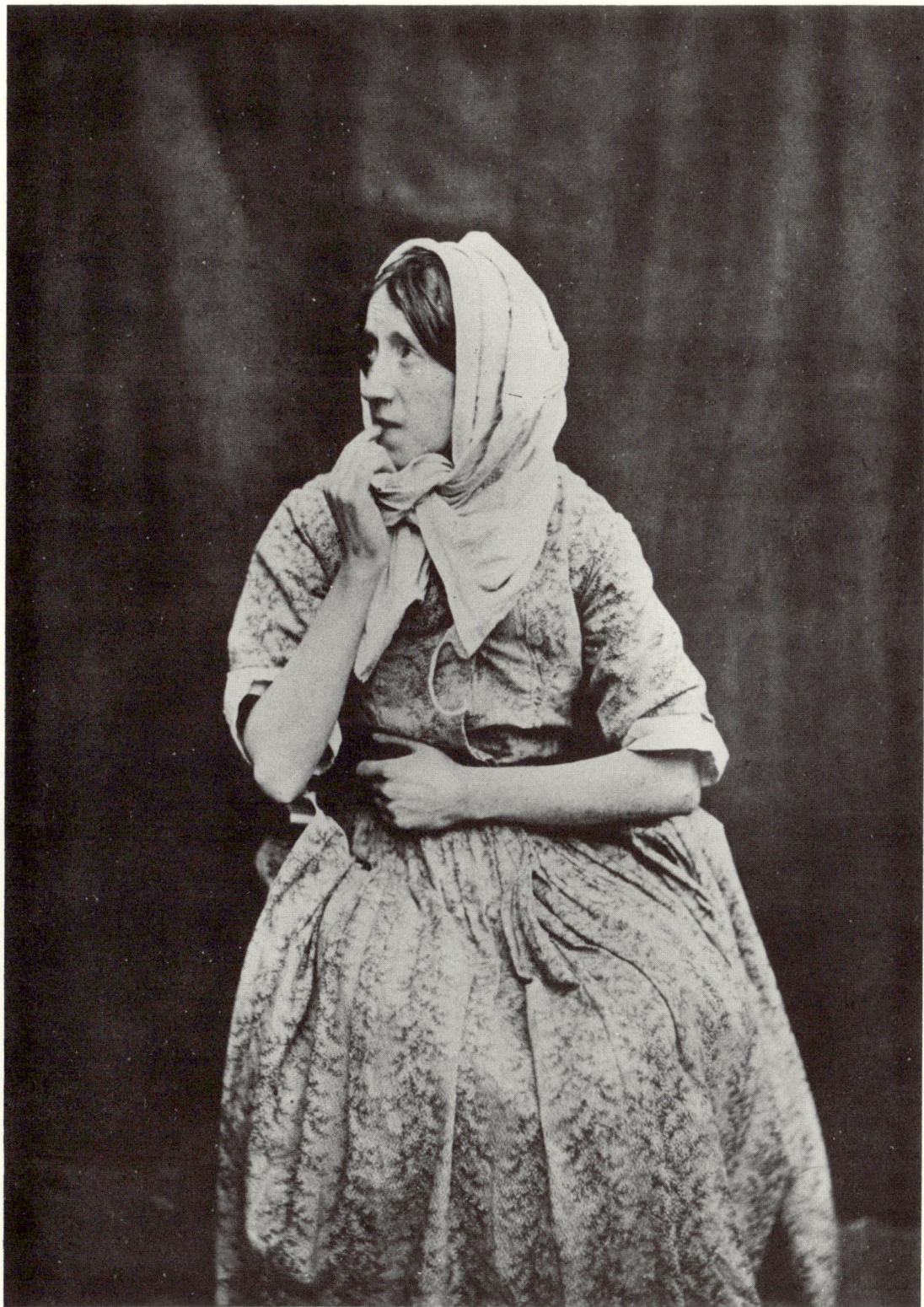

PLATE 25

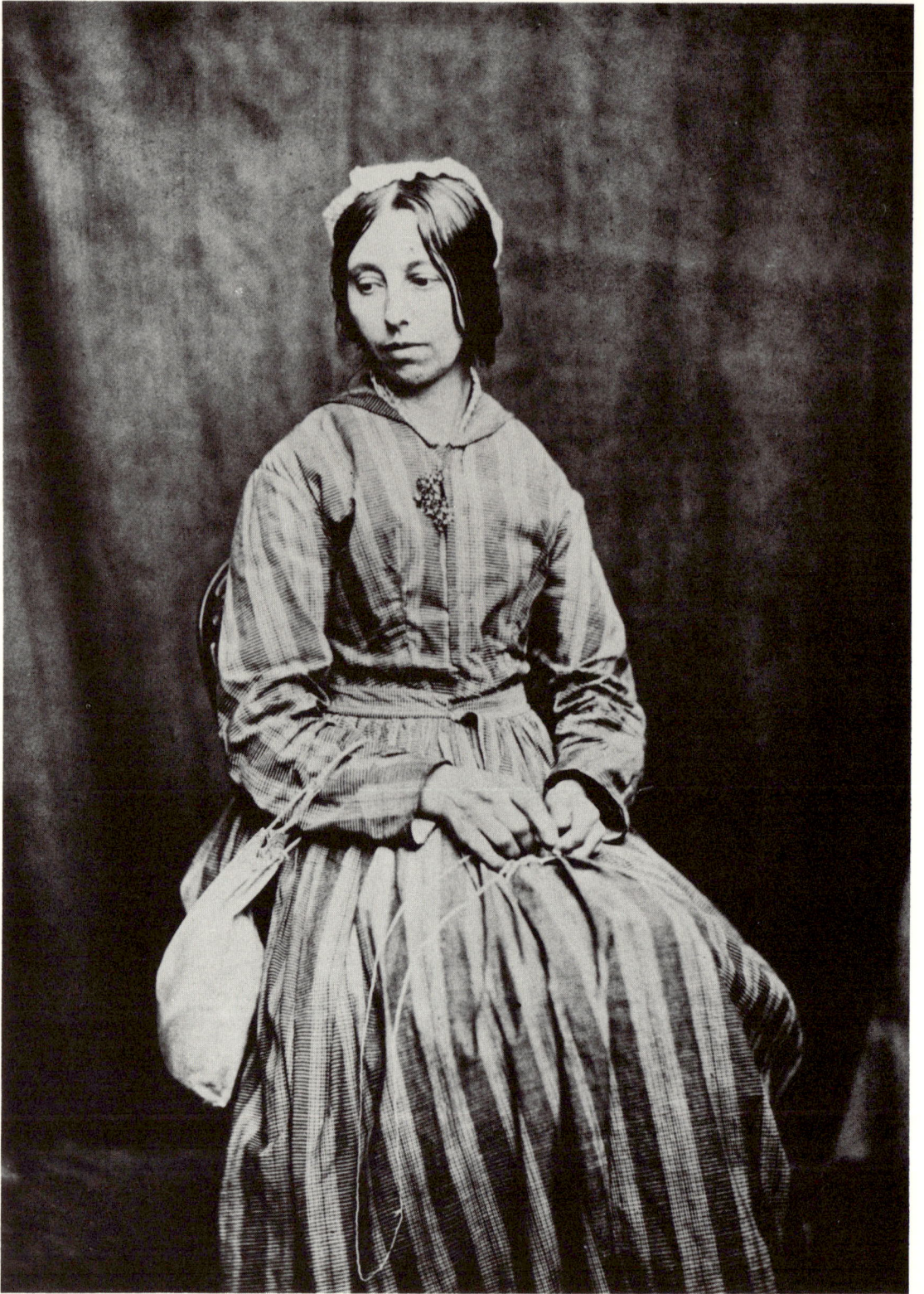

PLATE 26

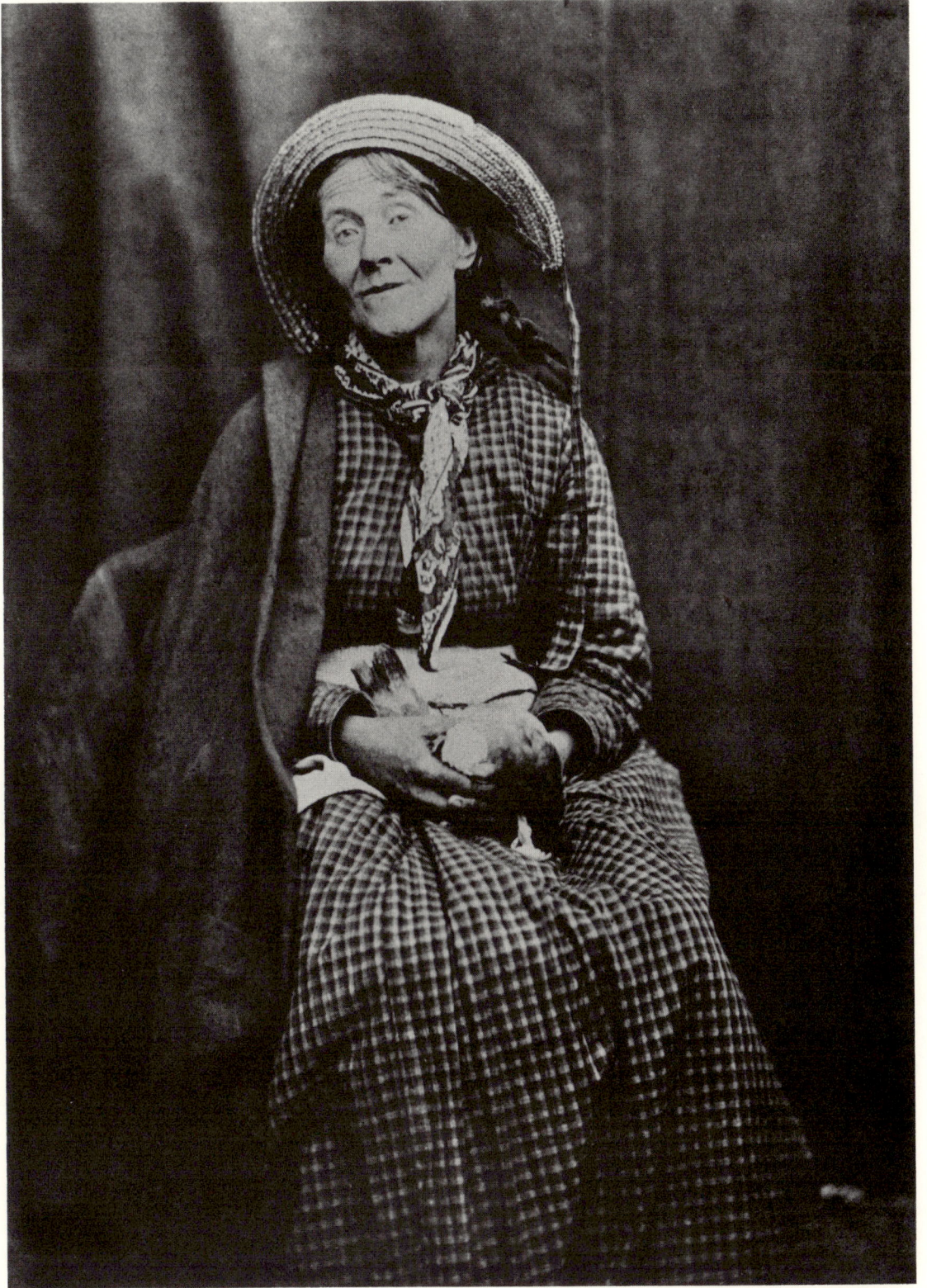

PLATE 27

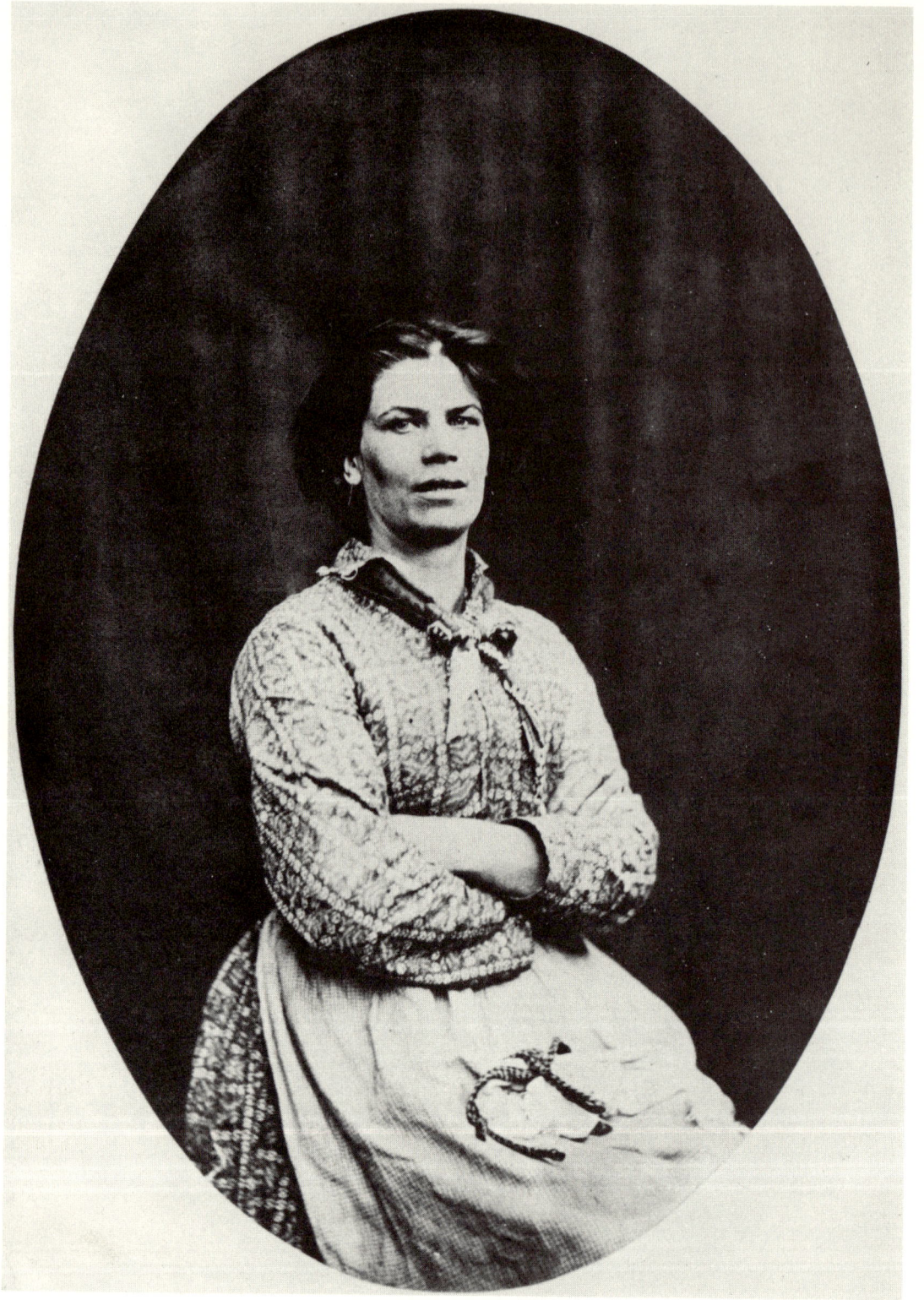

PLATE 28

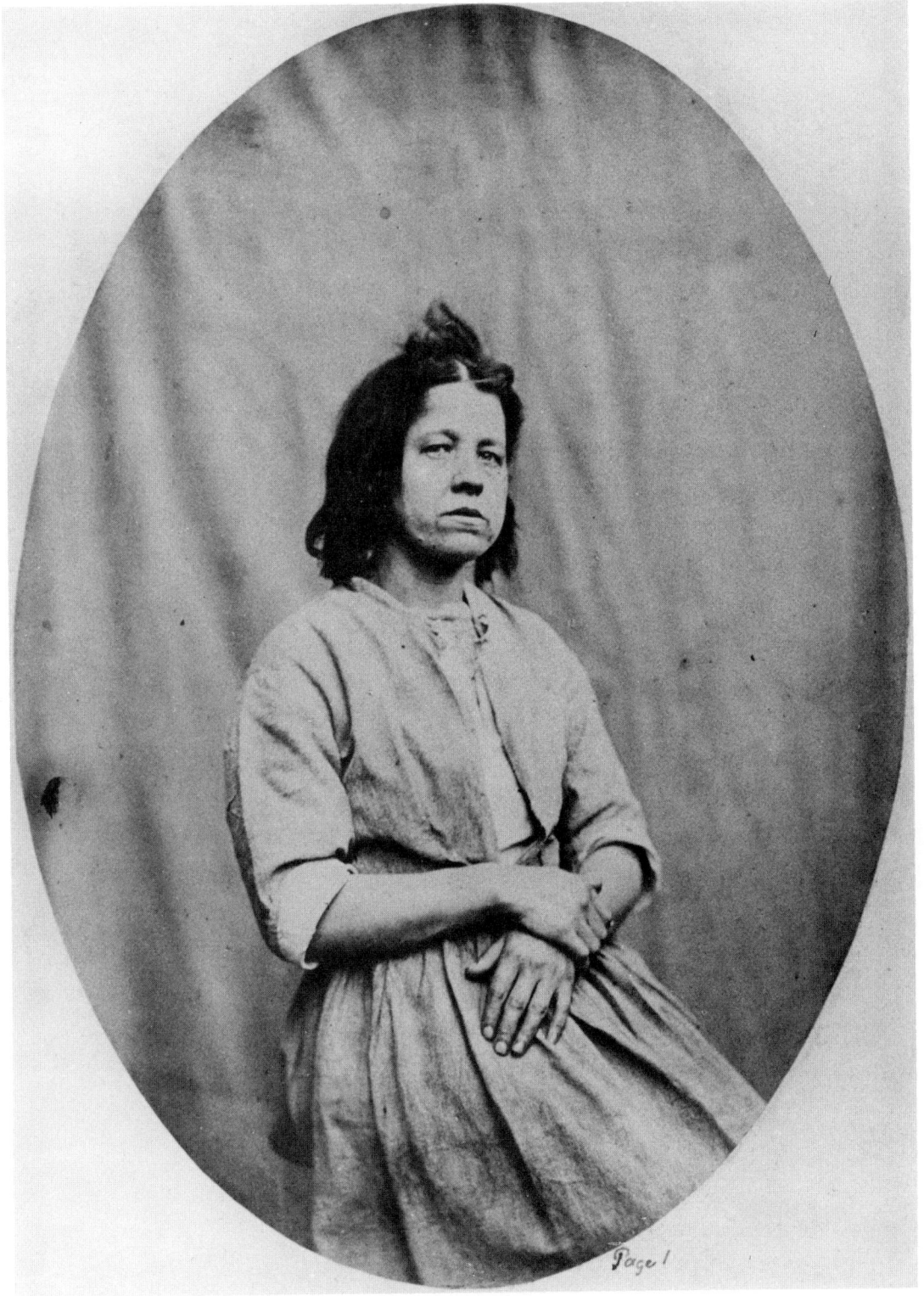

Page 1

PLATE 29

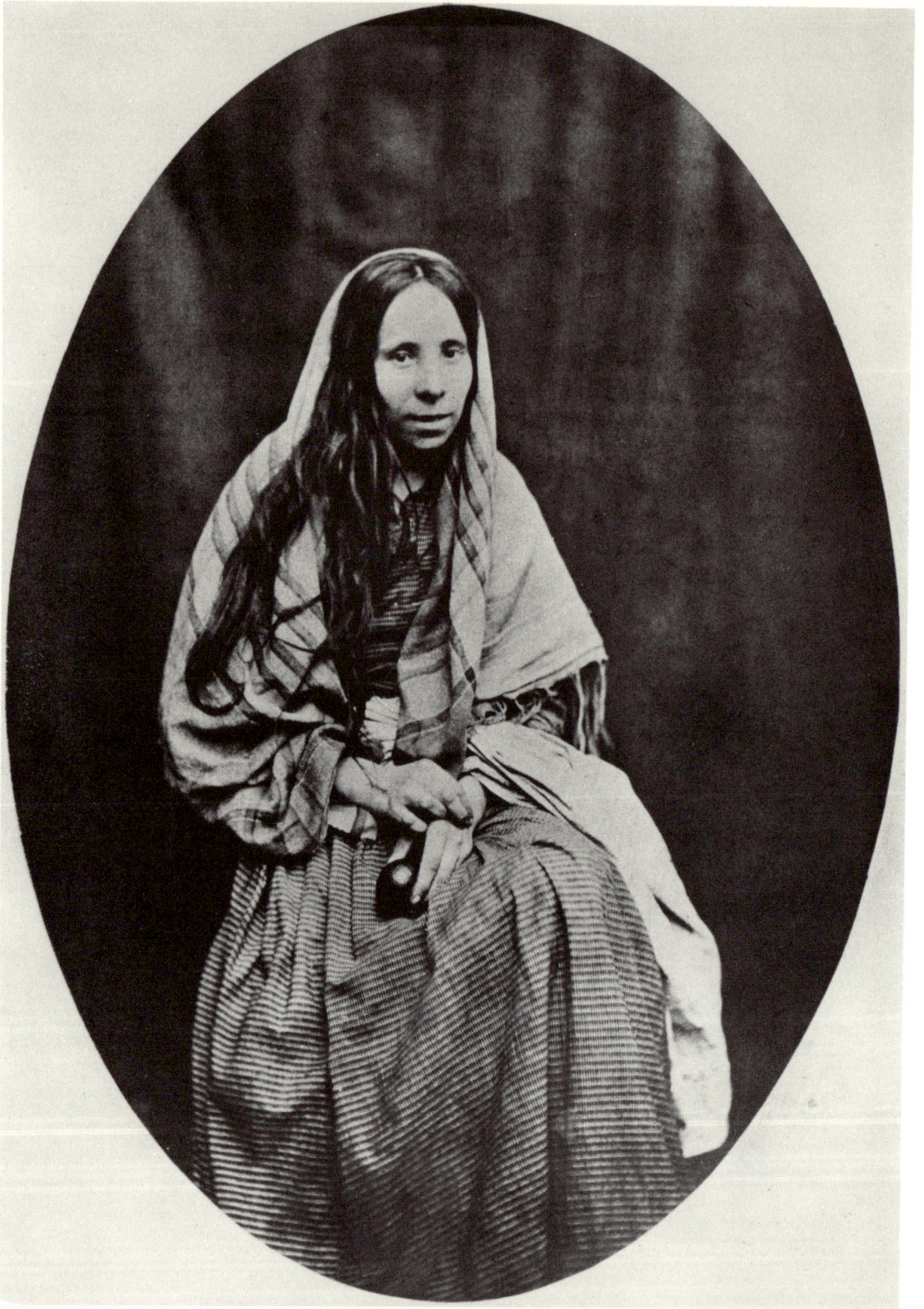

PLATE 30

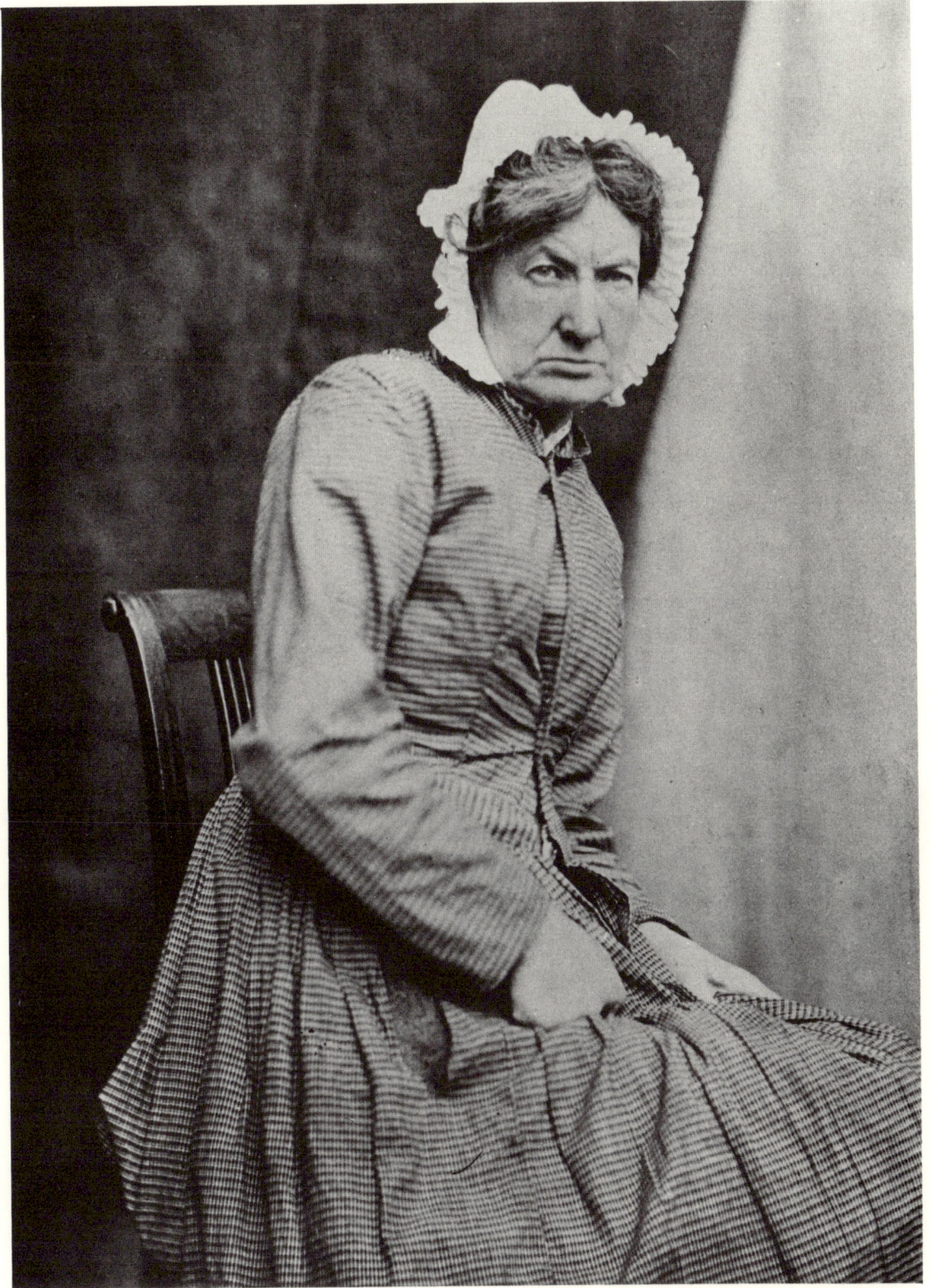

PLATE 31

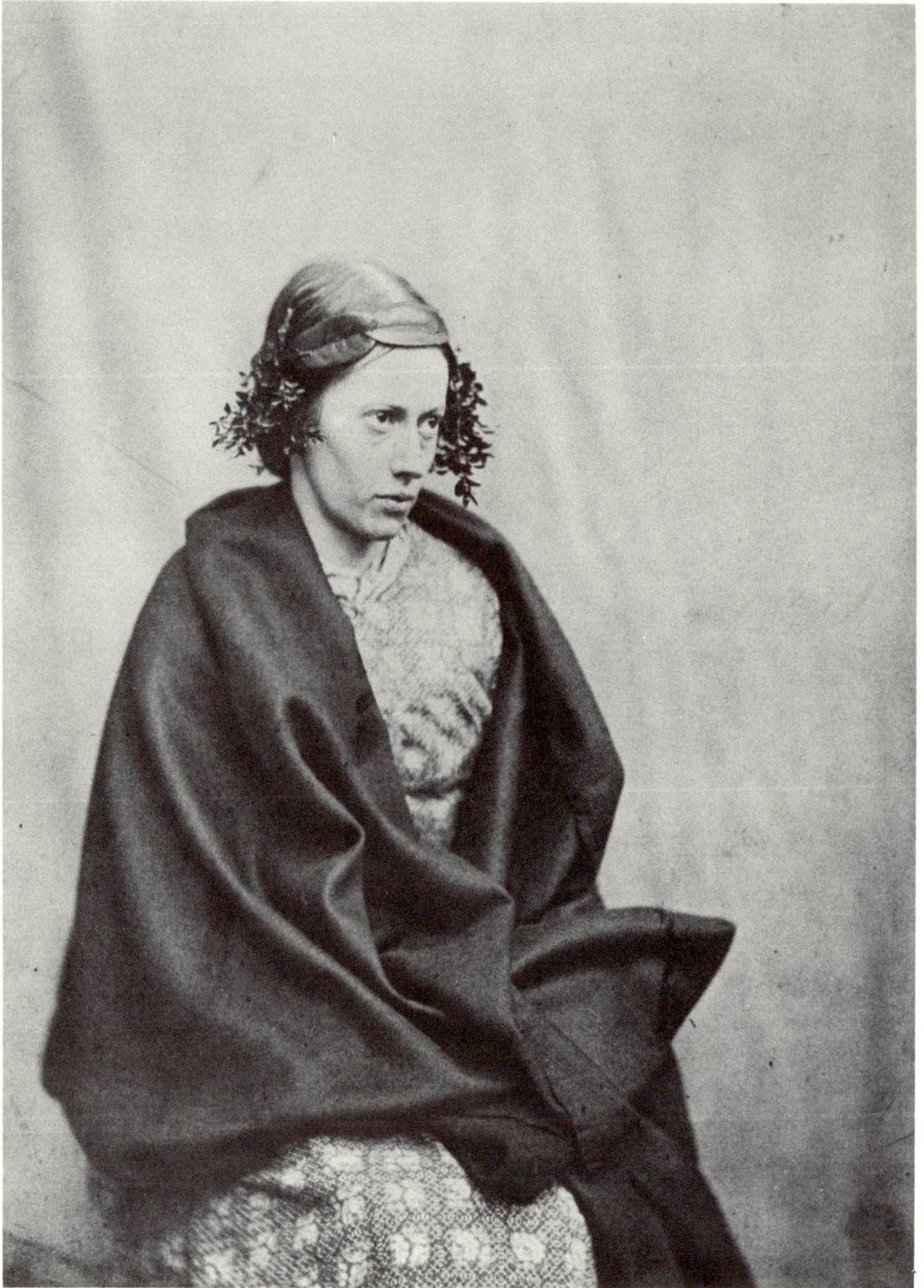

PLATE 32

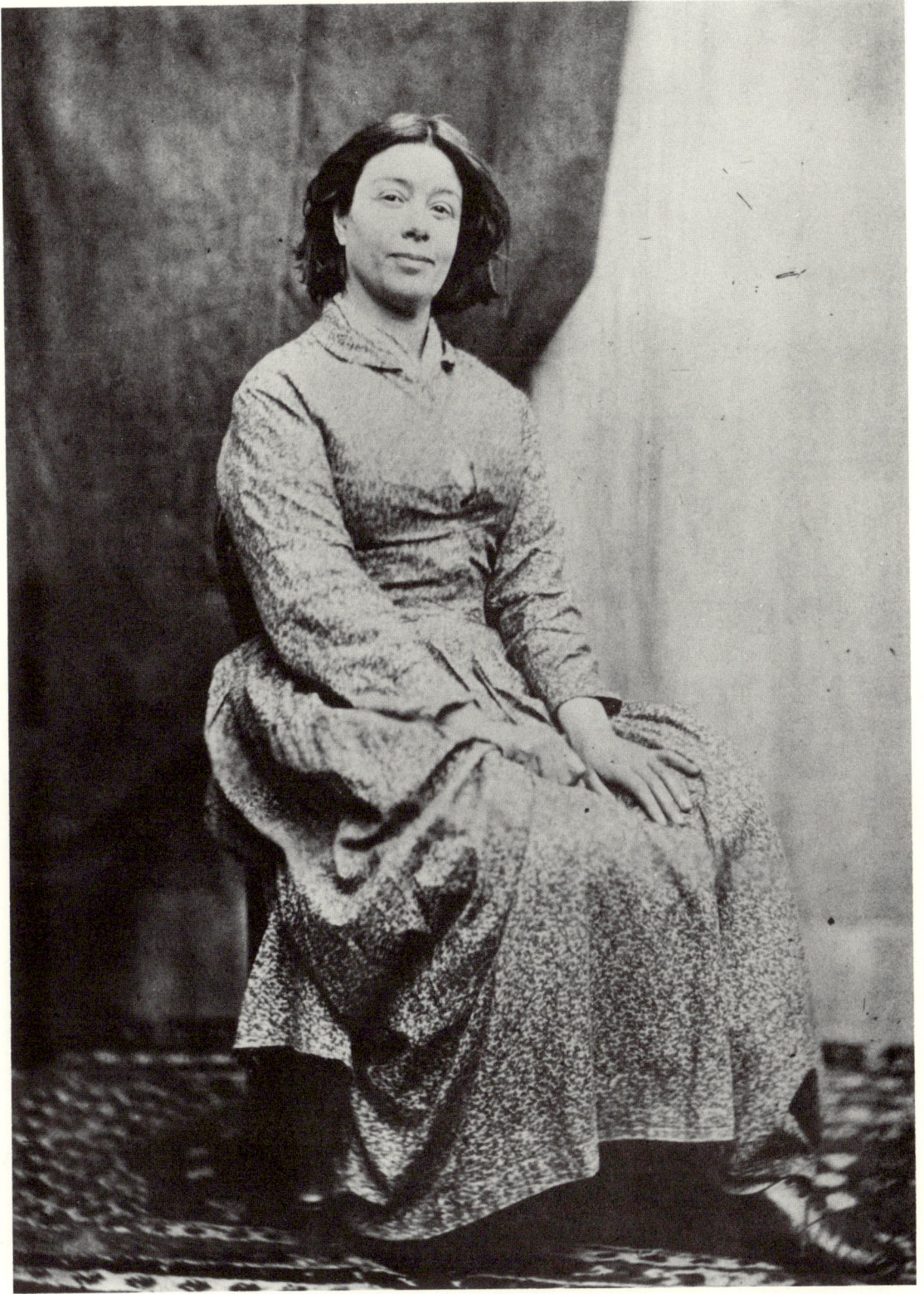

PLATE 33

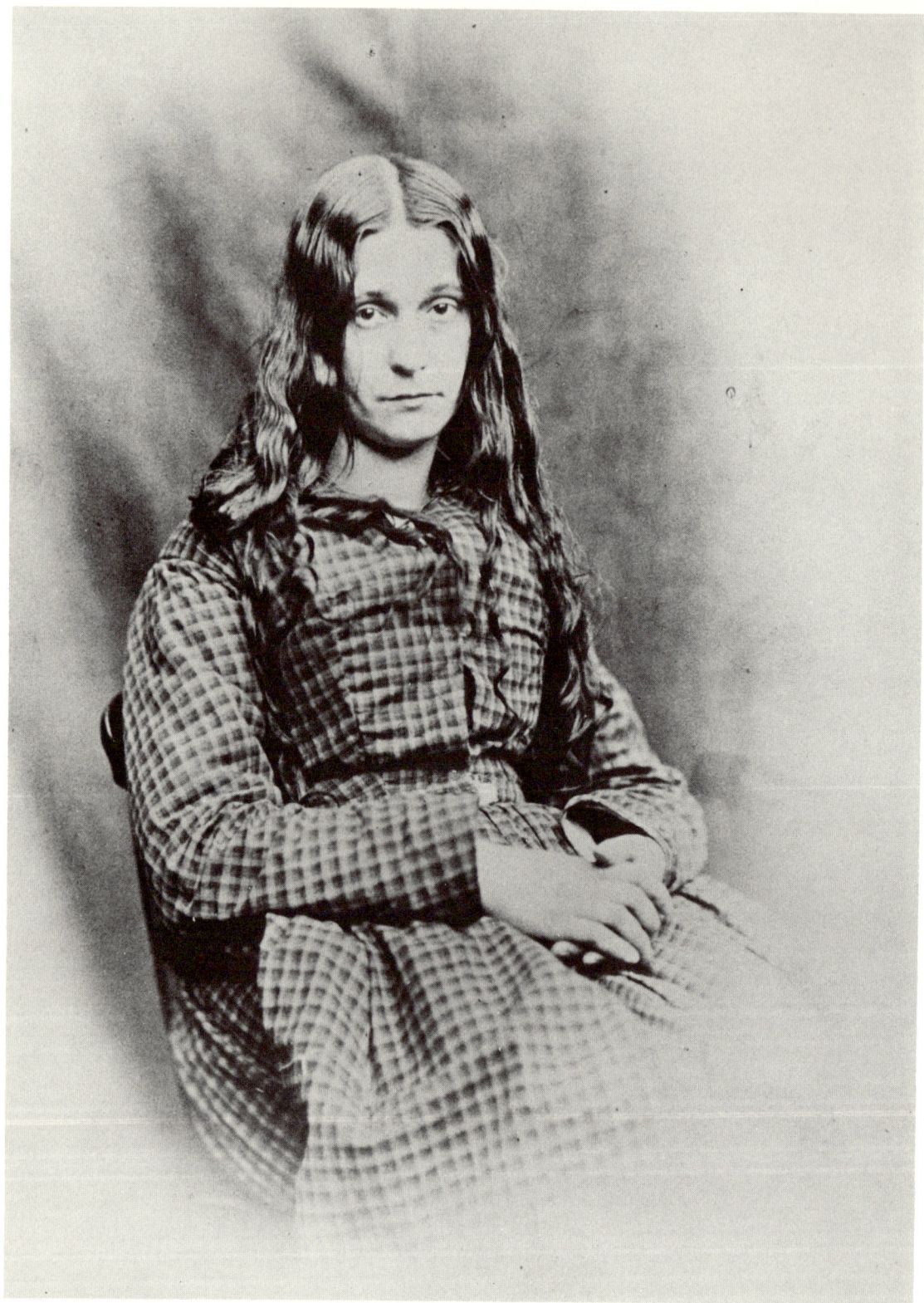

PLATE 34

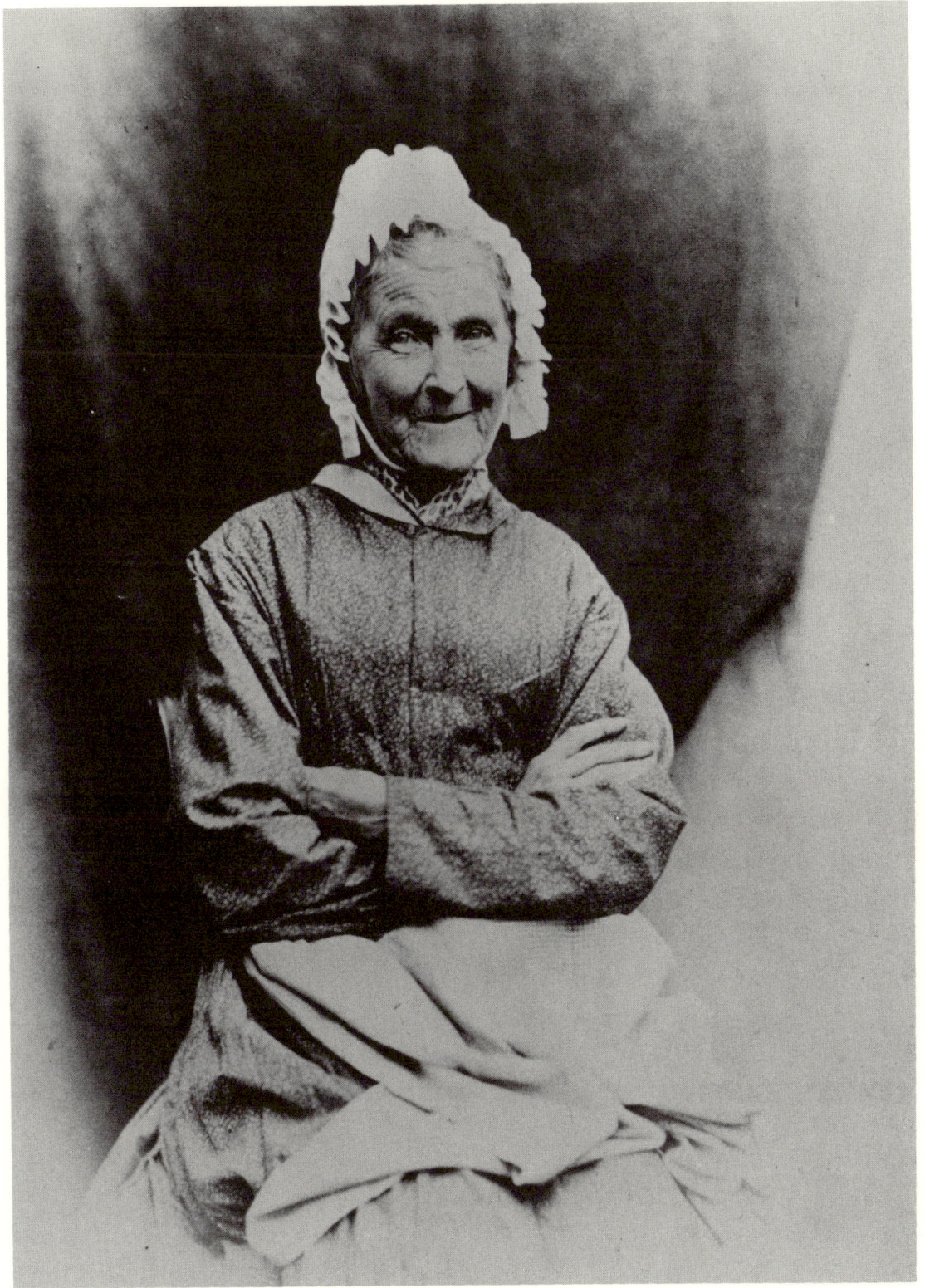

PLATE 35

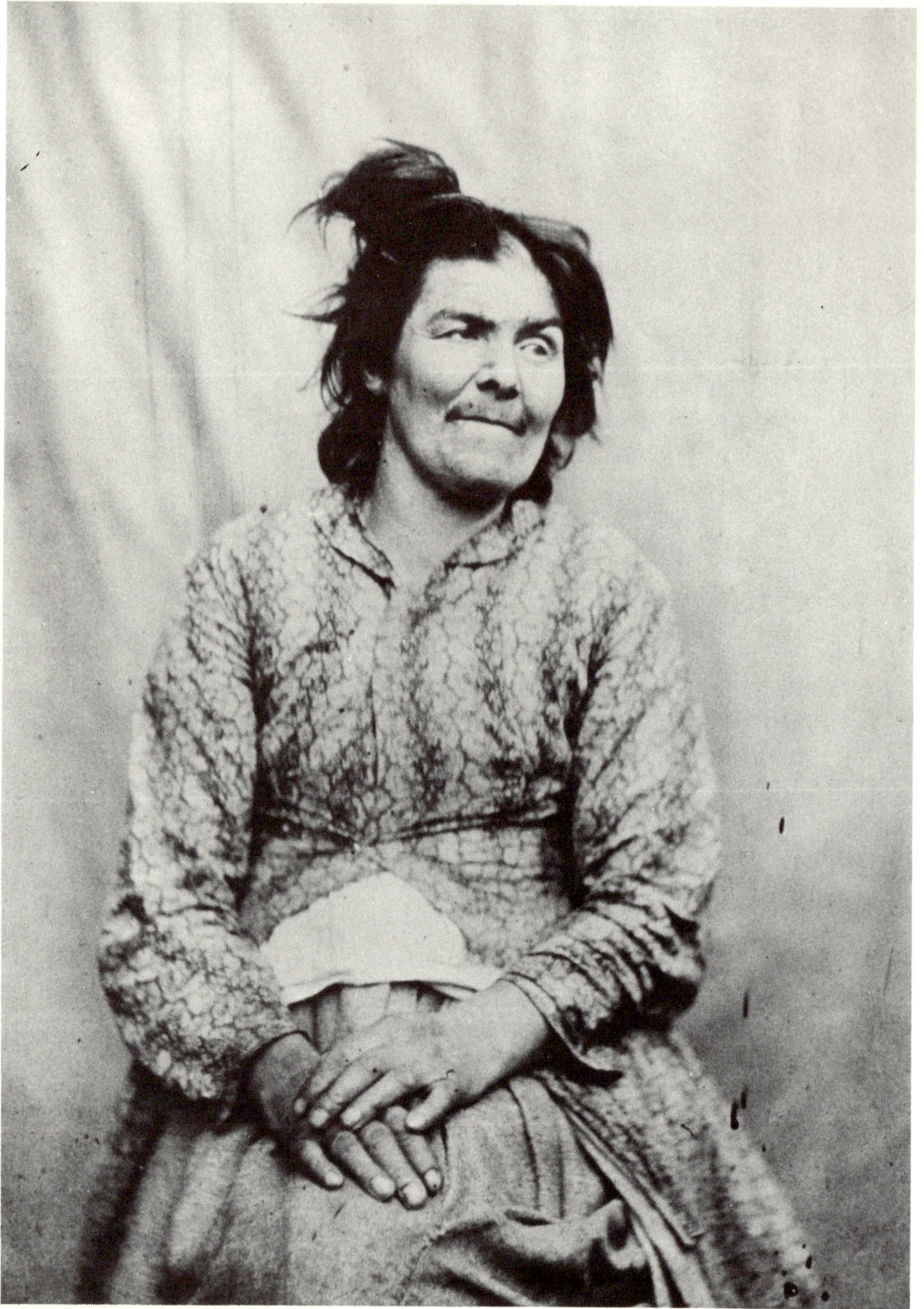

PLATE 36

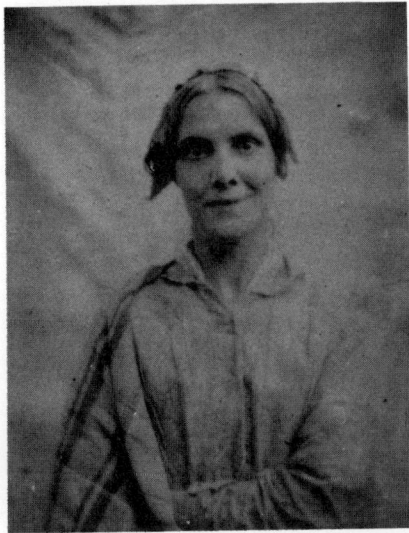

PLATE 37

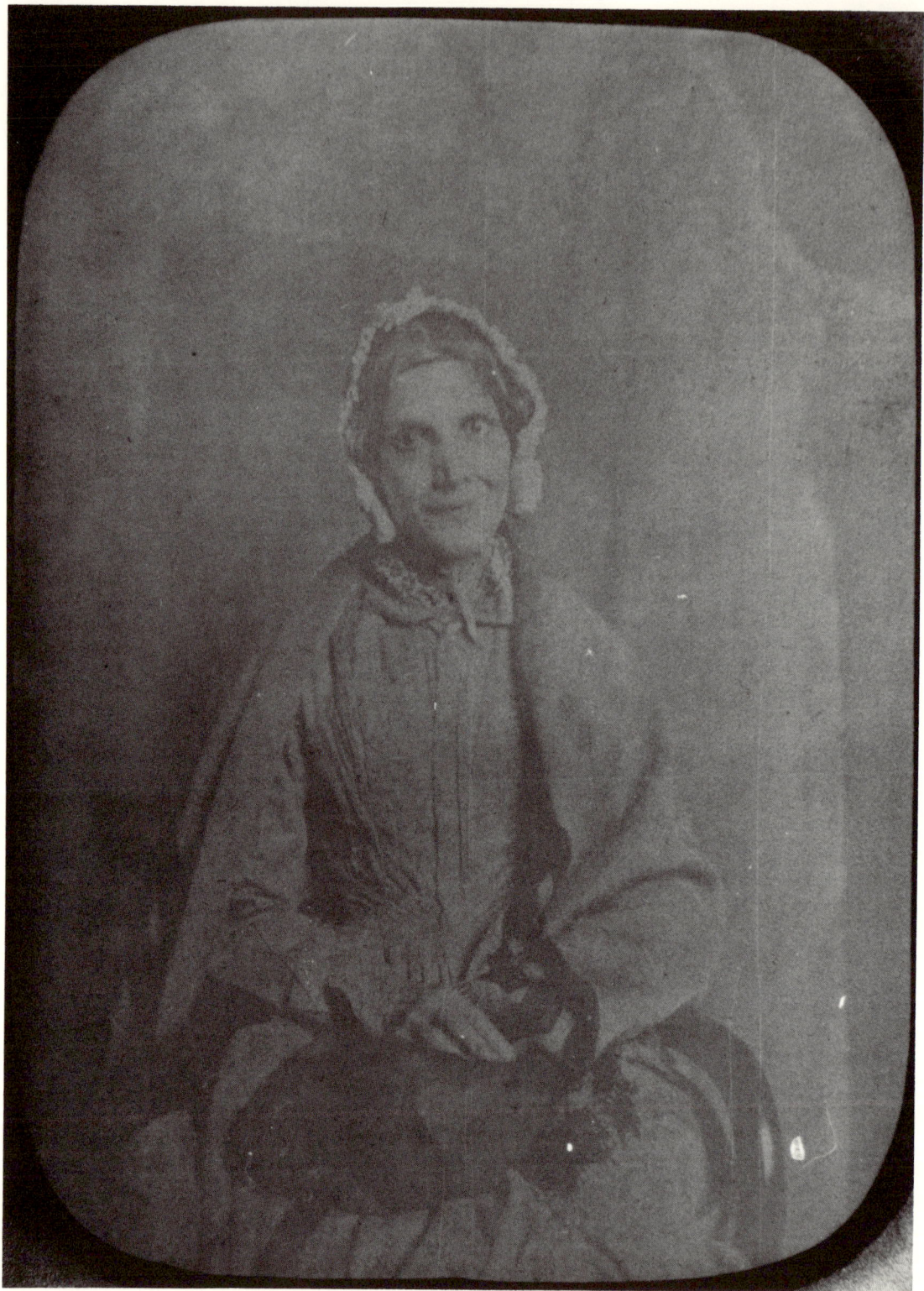

PLATE 38

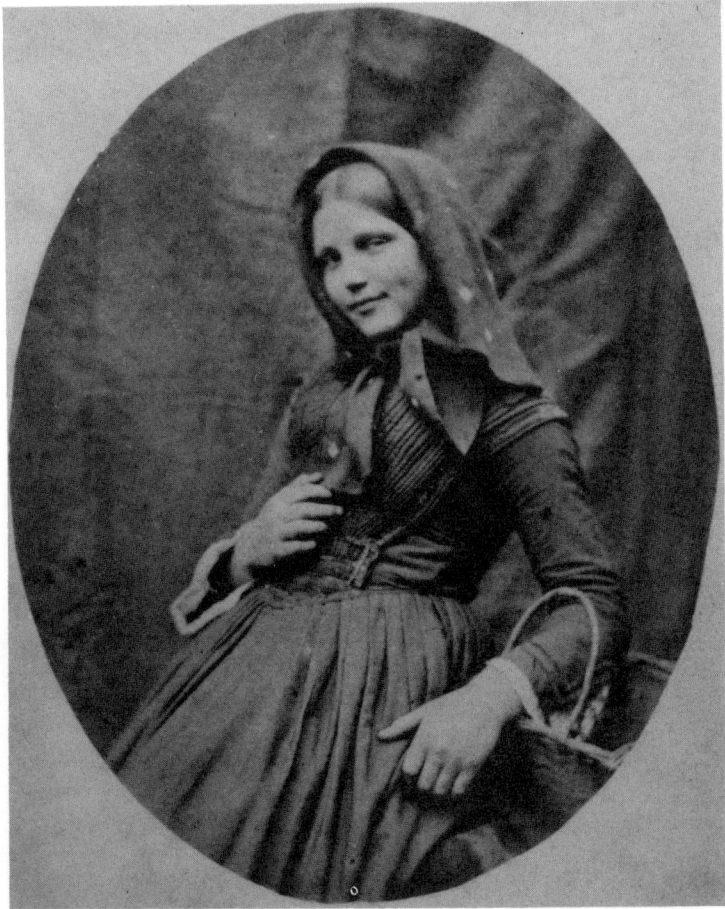

PLATE 39

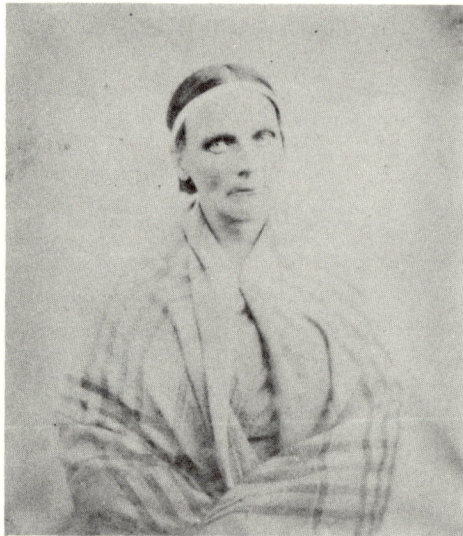

PLATE 40

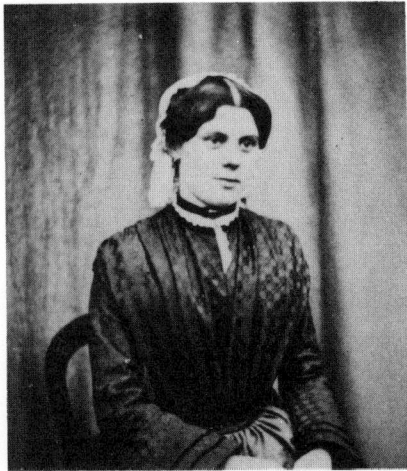

PLATE 41

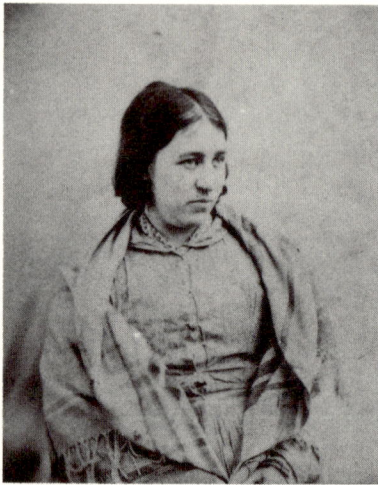

PLATE 42

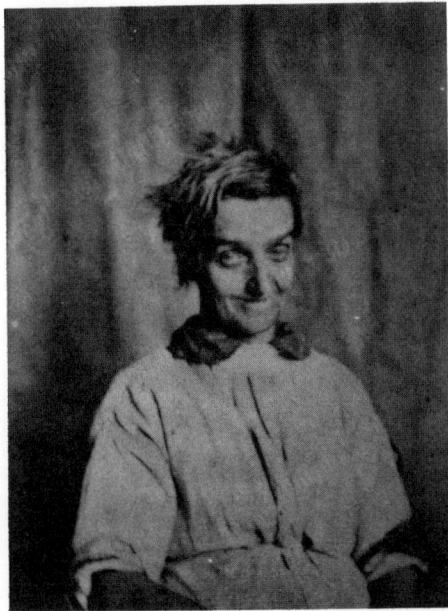

PLATE 43

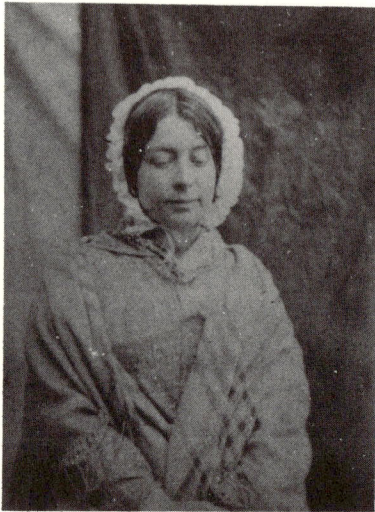

PLATE 44

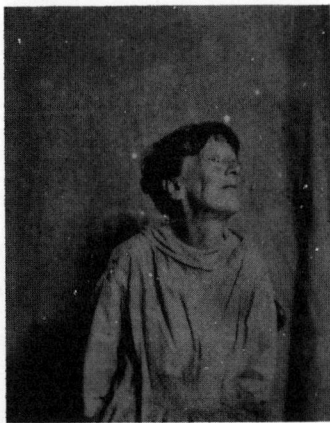

PLATE 45

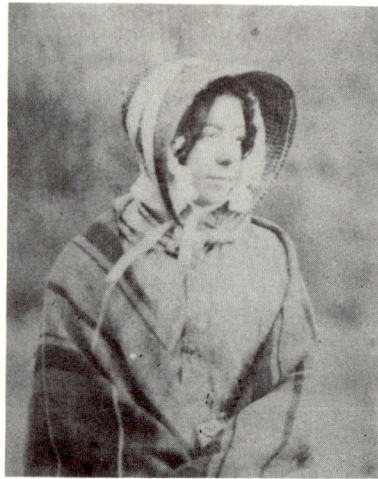

PLATE 46

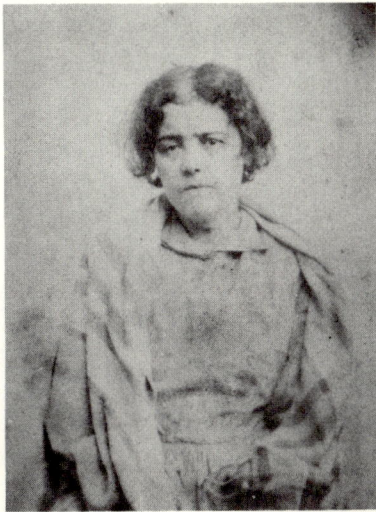

PLATE 47

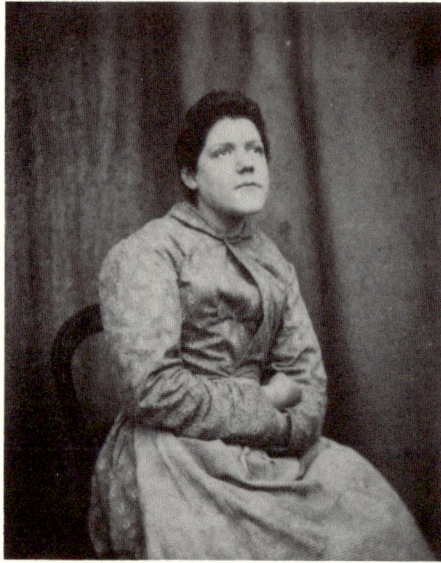

PLATE 48

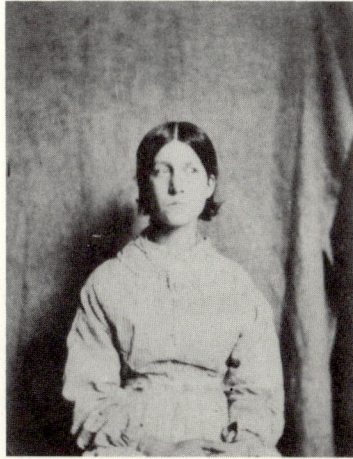

PLATE 49

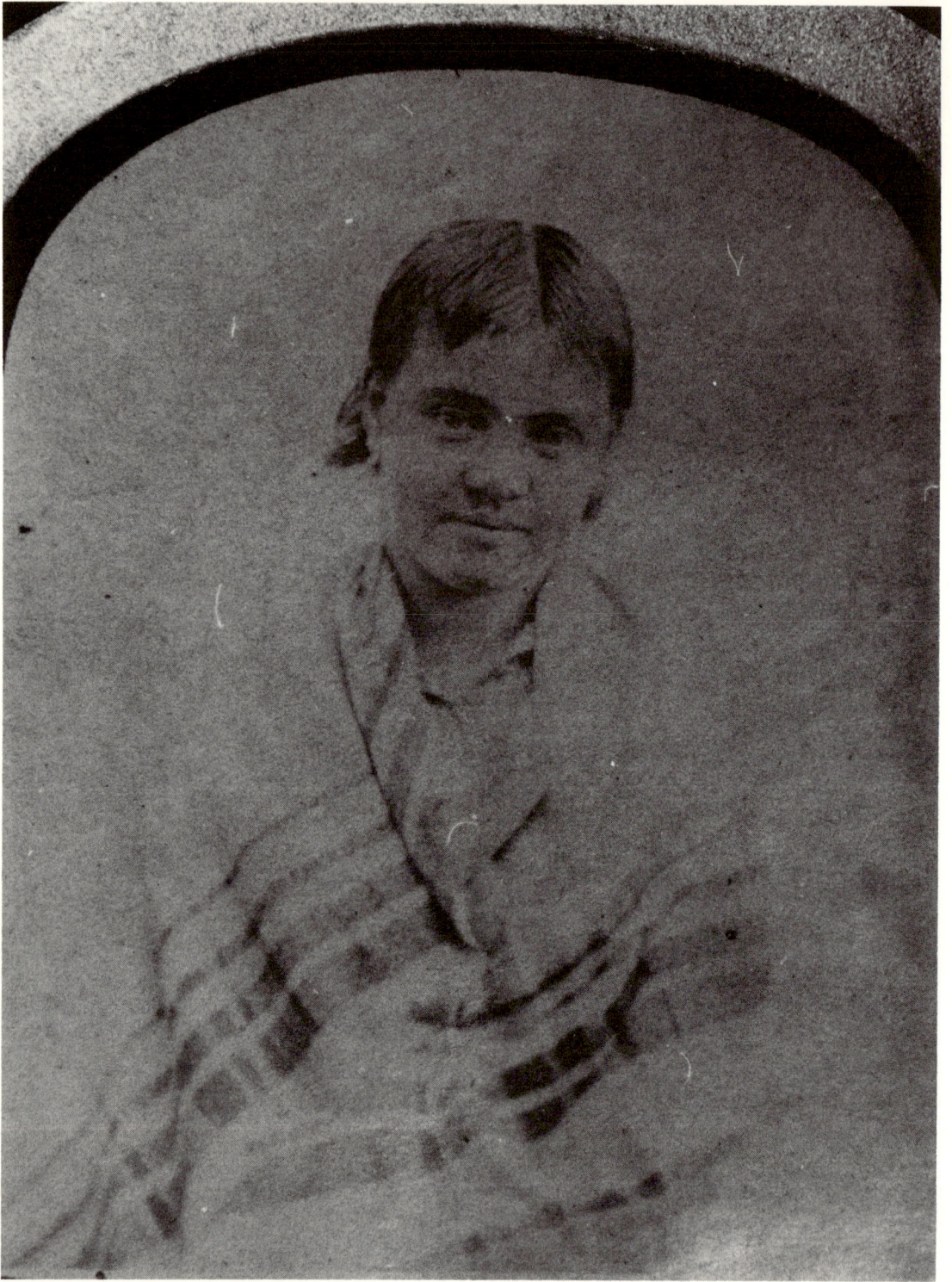

PLATE 50

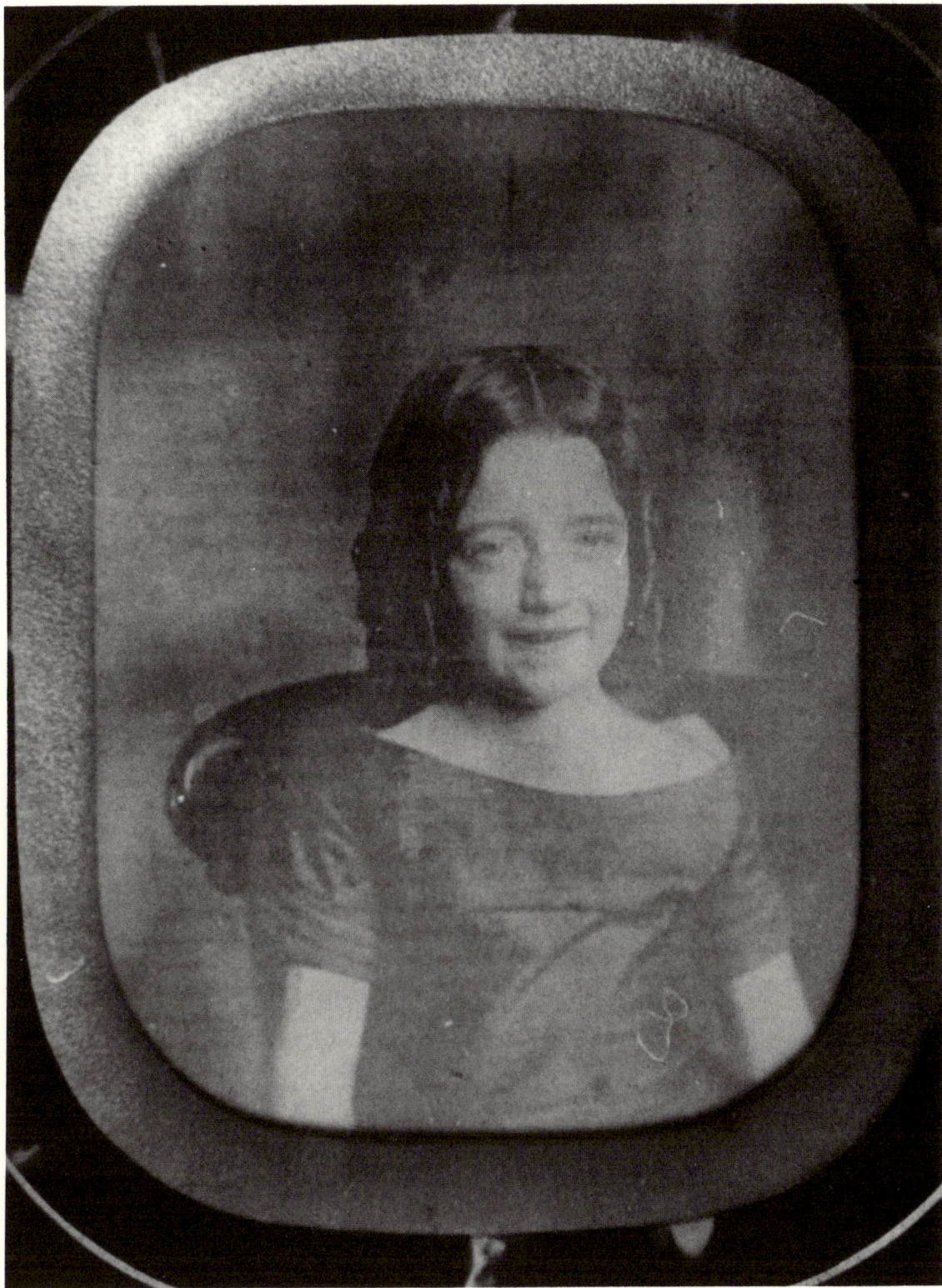

PLATE 51

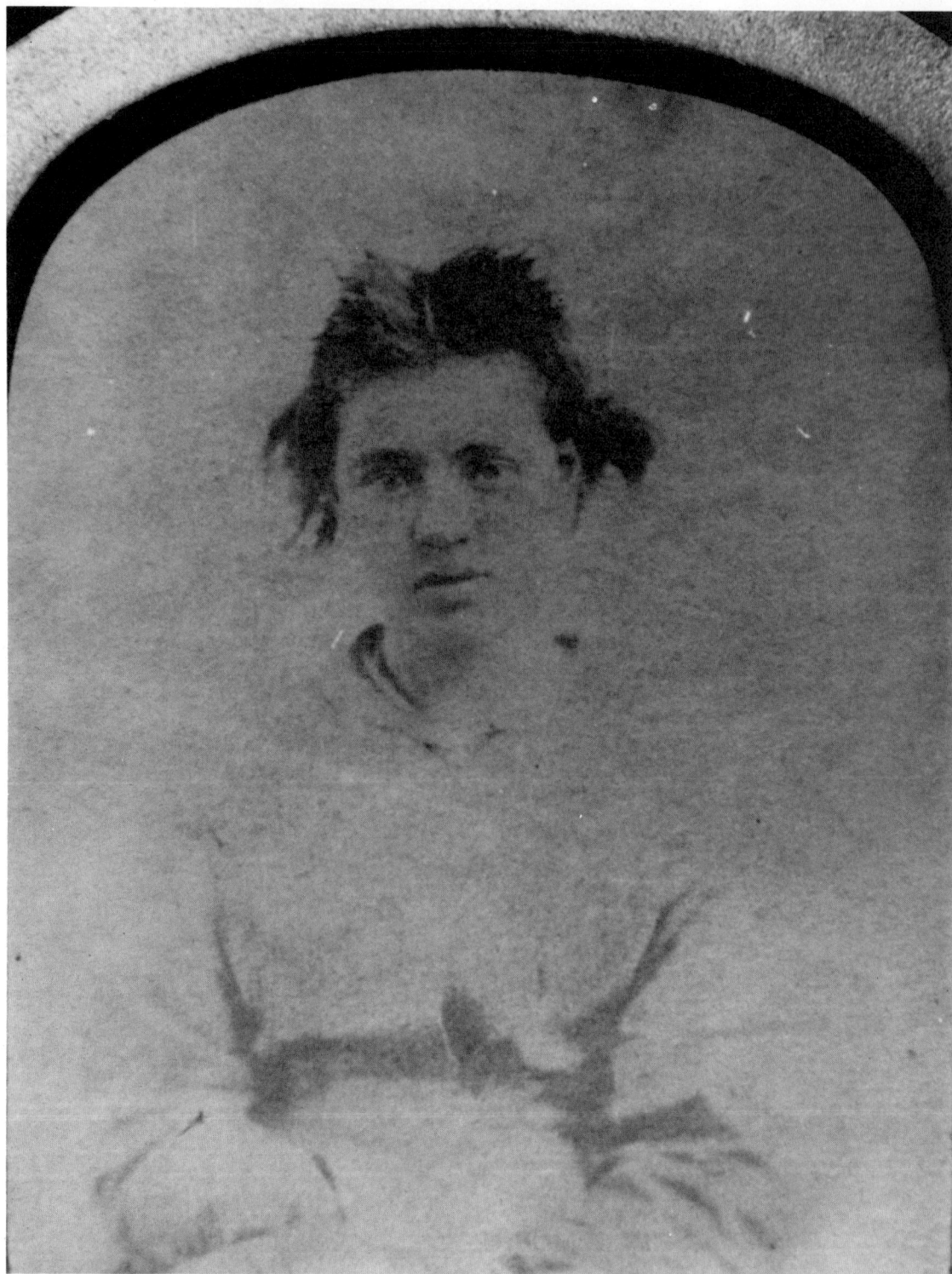

PLATE 52

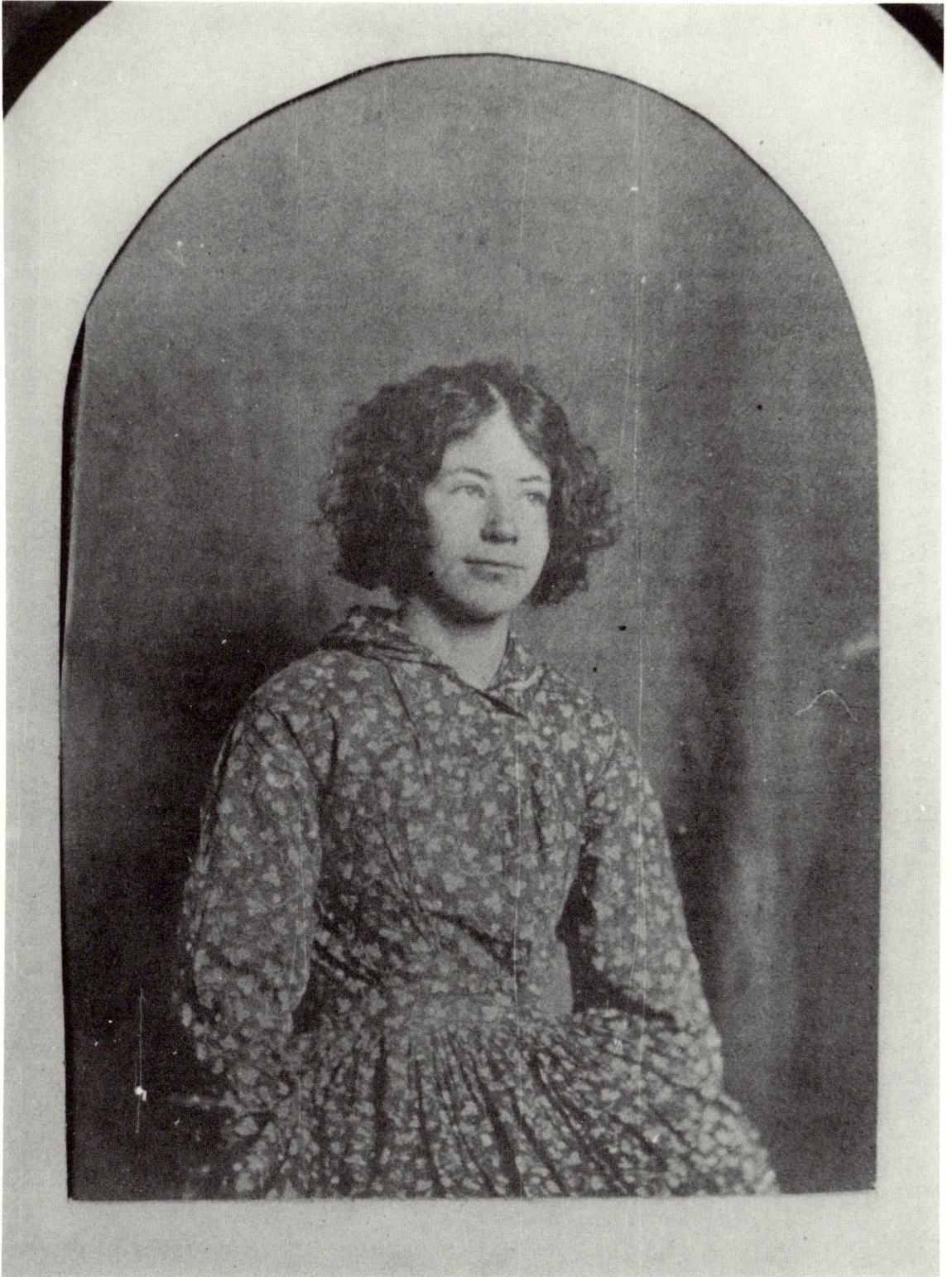

PLATE 53

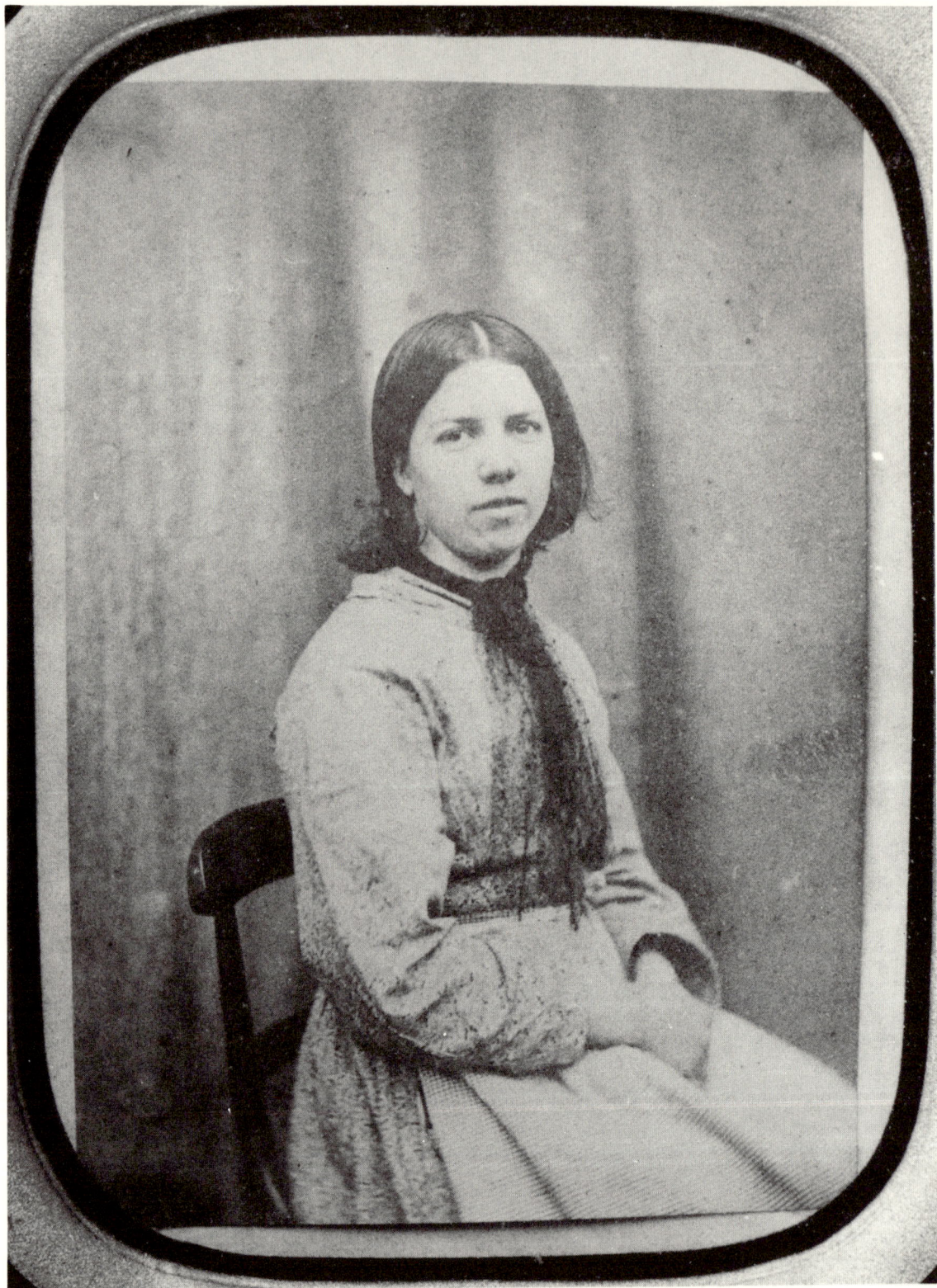

PLATE 54

PHOTOGRAPHIC SOURCES

Plates 1, 3, 5, 12, 16, 17, 18, 19, 20, 22, 24, 25, 26, 27, 28, 29, 30, 31, 32, 33, 34, 35, 36, are reproduced with the permission of the Royal Society of Medicine (London).

Plates 2, 4, 6, 9, 11, 13, 14, 15, are reproduced from *The Medical Times and Gazette* (1858).

Plates 7, 8, 21, 23, 37, 39, 40, 41, 42, 43, 44, 45, 46, 47, 48, 49, are reproduced with the permission of the Royal Photographic Society (London).

Plates 10, 38, 50, 51, 52, 53, 54, are reproduced with the permission of the Norfolk Record Office (Norwich).